On the Brink:

The Inside Story of Fukushima Daiichi

On the Brink:
The Inside Story
of
Fukushima Daiichi

by

Ryūshō Kadota

Translation: **Simon Varnam**

Technical supervision: **Akira Tokuhiro**

Kurodahan Press
2014

On the Brink: The Inside Story of Fukushima Daiichi

ISBN 978-4-902075-54-0
NG-JP0043A3

Text for this edition was prepared for publication with the assistance of Proof Perfect Editorial Services and Milo Barisof.

KURODAHAN.COM

Contents

Northern Japan

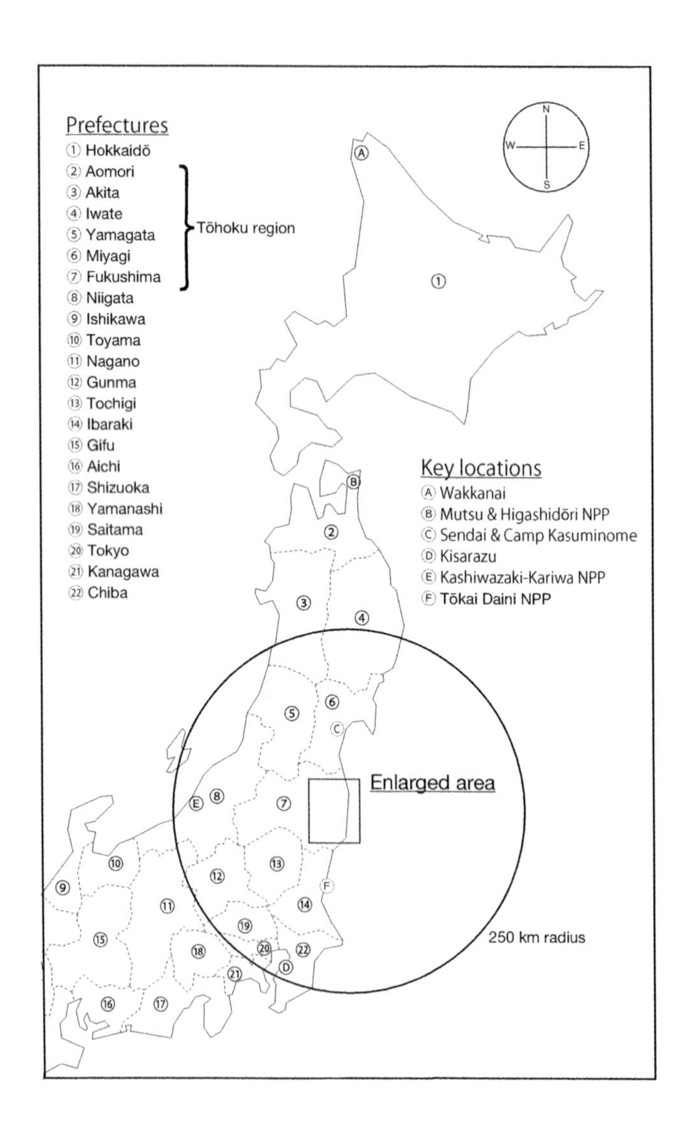

The Fukushima Region

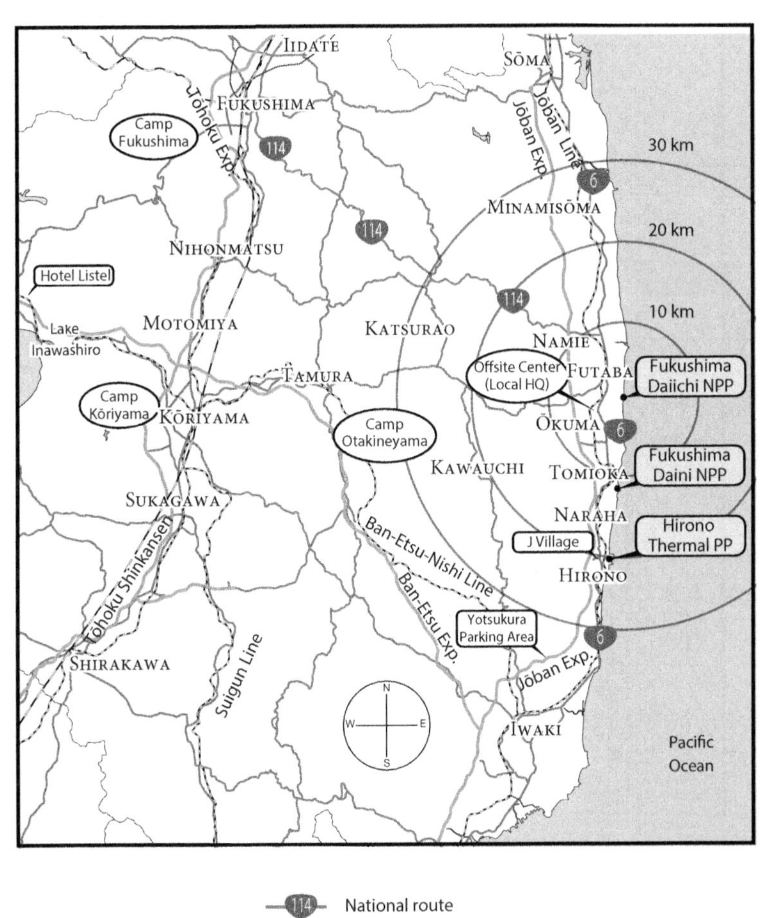

Fukushima Daiichi Layout

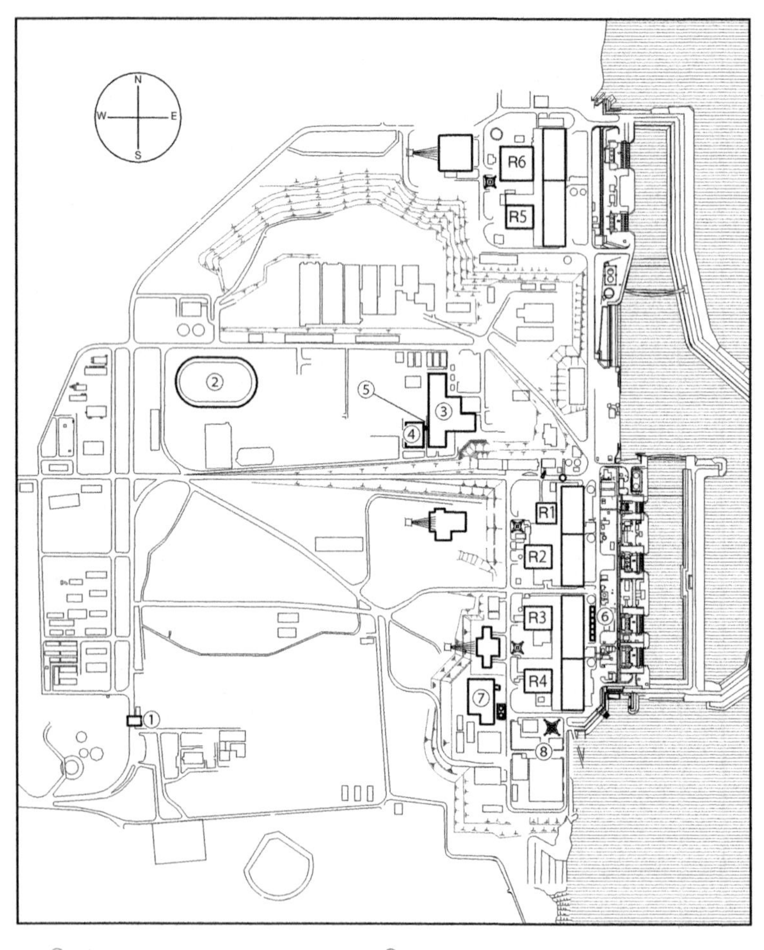

①	Main gate	⑤	Connecting link
②	Sports field	⑥	Reversing valve pit No. 3
③	Administration building	⑦	Auxiliary services building
④	Quakeproof building (QPB)	⑧	Camera (see page 27)

Cutaway view of reactor assembly (Unit 1)

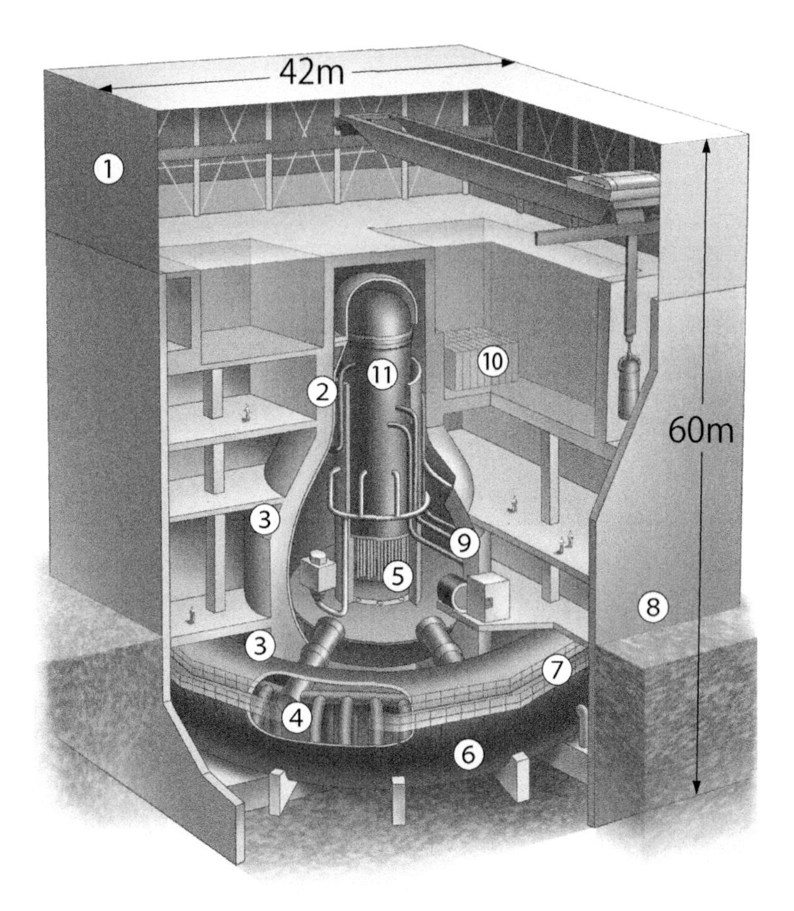

①	Fifth floor: blown off by explosion	⑥	Suppression chamber torus
②	Concrete primary containment vessel	⑦	Catwalk
③	Approximate locations of valves opened during incursions	⑧	Ground floor entrance, ten meters above sea level
④	Vent pipes	⑨	Pipes used to inject water
⑤	Control rods	⑩	Spent fuel rods in pool
		⑪	Reactor pressure vessel

N.B. For clarity, this diagram is greatly simplified and not strictly to scale. Many of the 'empty' spaces are actually crammed with piping, wiring, access ladders, and miscellaneous equipment.

Fukushima Daiichi, Units 1–4

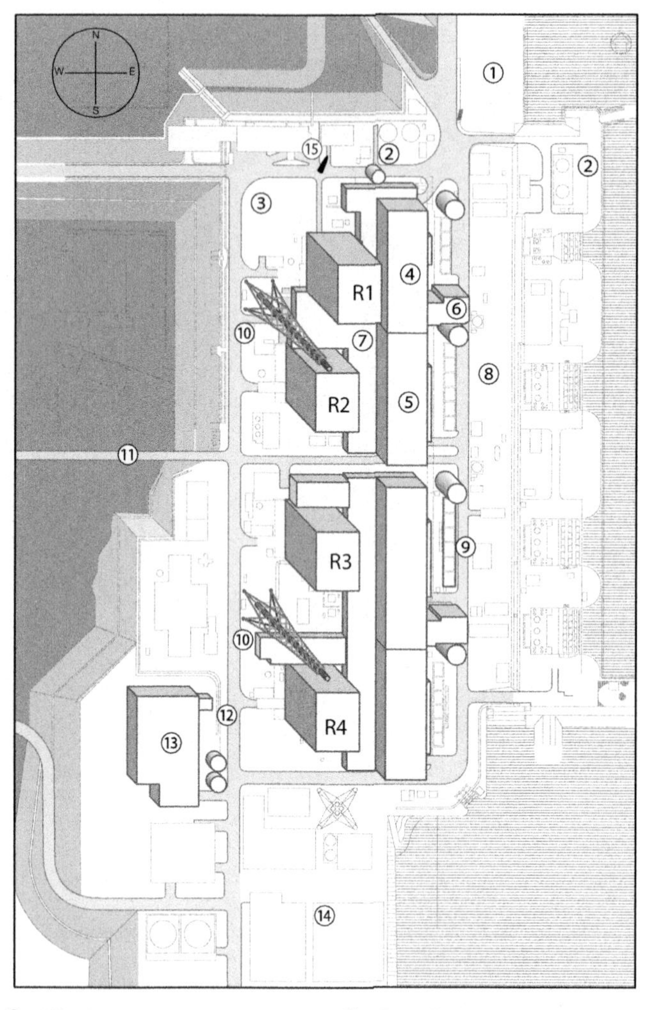

① Wharf
② Oil tank (before and after)
③ 10-meter level
④ Turbine building No. 1
⑤ Turbine building No. 2
⑥ Service building
⑦ Control room 1 & 2 (below)
⑧ 4-meter level
⑨ Reversing valve pit No. 3
⑩ Ventilation stack
⑪ Route used by fire engines
⑫ Site of Iga and Ara's escape
⑬ Auxiliary services building
⑭ Camera (see page 27)
⑮ Boat washed ashore

Fukushima Daiichi Flooding

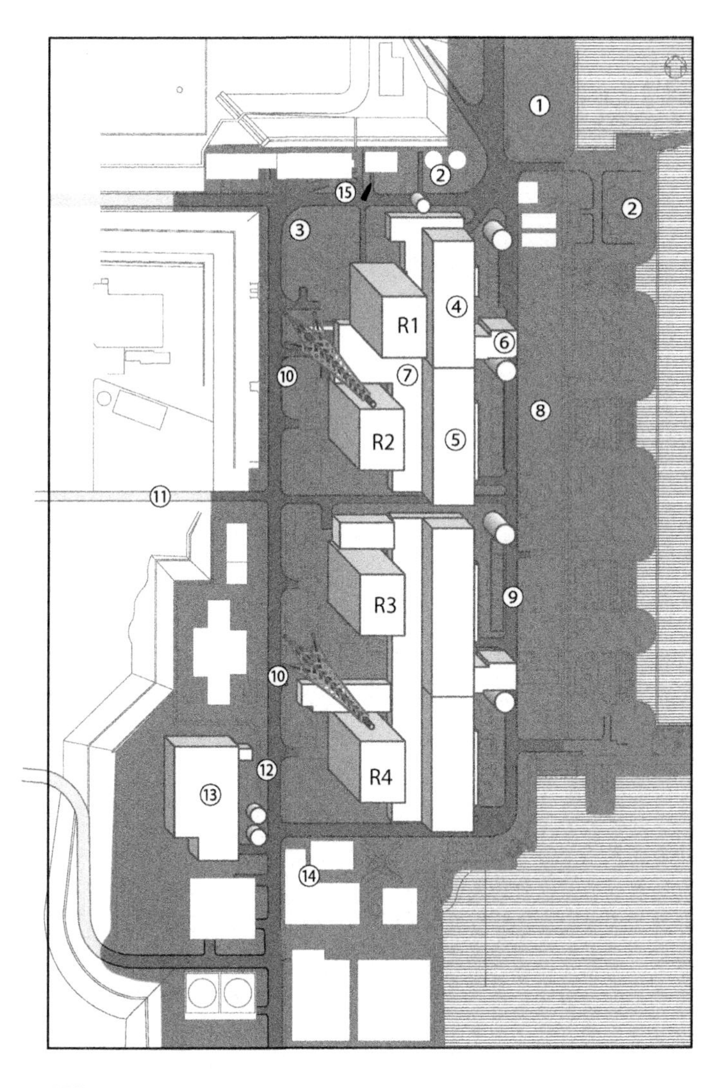

Flooded area

Acknowledgements

THIS BOOK HAS COME to fruition only through the efforts of a huge number of people.

Starting with Masao Yoshida, Site Superintendent at FDI, I must also mention the employees of TEPCO and contracted companies who labored on at the plant, the self-defense forces personnel who mobilized, the politicians and government officials who organized emergency responses, researchers, local journalists, evacuees, the relatives of those who died in the accident, and countless others whose kind contributions have enabled the completion of this book.

The truth of this unforeseen disaster must be passed on to future generations.

This was the common goal of all the contributors. It was only the enthusiasm of these generous souls that pushed me on and enabled me to overcome the numerous trials and tribulations of completing the book.

During the interview process, I discovered unexpected difficulties and moving human drama largely unknown to the world.

While penning this documentary, I keenly felt that there are times when people have to risk their lives.

The men who made the incursions into the reactor building had families. If these breadwinners had died, their families would have been left destitute, with their futures in doubt.

Nevertheless, they resolved to act. The soldiers, too, though the accident was none of their doing, ignored the danger to their own lives and carried out their missions in the radiation-contaminated area.

The thing that surprised me most when I interviewed them about their roles was that they regarded the work as a matter of course, and even now wouldn't dream of being so vain as to brag about the experience. In fact, though they were among the first responders, bringing their fire engines to initiate recovery of the plant, they themselves were surprised that I should come specially to talk with them about it.

"We only did what was expected of us. I doubt that many, even in the forces, have even heard about the operation we carried out there."

The TEPCO employees at the plant and the people working for contracted companies too, the people who carried on working as radiation levels rose; all had the same kind of attitude toward their work, something which I found both surprising and deeply moving.

I have written a number of books related to the Pacific War. In them, I have referred to the generation that supplied the main fighting strength of the nation – the generation born in the Taishō era (1912-26) – and which suffered more than two million dead, as 'the generation that lived for others.' In contrast, I have criticized the current generation as one that lives for itself alone.

However, one unexpected thing that the tragedy of this nuclear accident has taught me is that the people of Japan retain the same sense of dedication and responsibility as their forebears, facing their problems with resolution, even to the point of risking their lives.

Besides the reality of the tragedy of this nuclear catastrophe, I hope this book has also shown the true power and conviction that people in desperate circumstances can find in the eleventh hour.

A question that occupied me throughout the collection of material for this book was how they were able to push themselves so far. I will be delighted if this book enables readers to find the answer to that question.

I must apologize for not naming all of the people who contributed to this book in so many ways; their number is huge. For the fact that this non-fiction book has reached publication, I offer my deepest thanks to all of them.

Ryūshō Kadota

Introduction

THE ACCIDENT AT FUKUSHIMA Daiichi has wrought unprecedented tragedy not only on Fukushima prefecture but on the whole of the northeastern Tōhoku region of Japan, while the aftereffects drag on even now, a year and a half after the earthquake. No one can say when the situation will be resolved.

People are anxious and angry. The sufferings of people who have had to abandon their hometowns, ordered to evacuate as if in wartime, and who still live in temporary housing or rented apartments, cannot be described with platitudes. Few find it easy to discuss their feelings on being forced to leave the land of their birth.

Fifteen months after the earthquake, Tokyo Electric Power Company (TEPCO), the company responsible for the accident, was effectively nationalized. It was already impossible for such a private enterprise to cover the enormous costs of compensation to the victims. Japan's largest power company, recognized as a symbol of Japan's prosperity, disappeared, to be reborn as a new company.

But within this series of events there was one aspect missing that I felt I simply had to know, and that was the human side of it all. In this, the most desperate situation imaginable, what actually happened on-site? How did they feel? How did they cope?

First they learned of a total power blackout, next an inoperative cooling system, rising radiation levels, and then hydrogen explosions — this kind of data coming in, minute by minute, must have banished all hope. With no way to cool the reactors they were on the verge of running amok, but many of the staff remained on-site to do what little they could. Though the news that reached the public was fragmented and infrequent, the image that we, the

Japanese public, got was that a few brave people had remained at the plant and were struggling to control the situation. The vision of people battling on in the darkness of a total blackout was beyond our imagination. We had a vague image of TEPCO employees, contractors' staff, even members of the military, who came and risked their lives – large numbers of people holding out in the midst of the radiation – but it was almost impossible to discern the human situation on site. Technical assessments and evaluations of the disaster have been issued since by independent bodies, by TEPCO, by the Diet (the Japanese Parliament) and by various government bodies, but none of them touches on the human aspect.

Soon after the accident, I started to approach TEPCO itself, the relevant government agencies, and local sources, in an attempt to pursue the matter, but there seemed to be a thick wall of silence that repeatedly rebuffed me. Though I struggled on with my research, it wasn't until the beginning of 2012 that a vague outline of the reality began to appear. I'd had a suspicion from the start, but the truth was far worse than I had imagined.

In the face of extreme adversity, people's strengths and weaknesses are exposed. Someone unremarkable may, at the moment of truth, reveal hidden strengths, while another who has always spoken noble words may, when it comes to the crunch, become a figure of shame.

In times of crisis, people reveal their true colors.

As time passed, I gradually gained glimpses of the truth of the matter. But I wasn't able to actually meet the man who had commanded on the frontline, Masao Yoshida, head of the Fukushima Daiichi nuclear power plant, until fifteen months after the accident.

"I thought the game was up, a number of times," Yoshida told me. "The situation we were in was like trying to land a plane with all the instruments blank and the controls knocked out. I have nothing but respect for all my staff, who risked their lives on the site there."

Since the accident, he had lost weight, having been hit with cancer and undergone an operation, and was now barely recognizable as his former self.

Despite his poor health, he had kindly endured two interviews with me totaling four and a half hours, but on July twenty-sixth,

2012, before I was able to conduct a third interview, the terrific stress and his fight with cancer weakened the blood vessels in his brain, leading to a hemorrhage requiring hospitalization and a further operation.

In addition to Yoshida, I was also able to repeatedly interview many of the people who had been with him there at FDI – TEPCO and contractor staff who were prepared to testify, military personnel, politicians, scientists, and local residents – a total of more than ninety in all.

At the time of the accident, the shift supervisors and on-duty staff for each of the six reactor units were in their respective control rooms, nestled between the units.

Though the detectors indicated high levels of radiation, and the alarms shrilled constantly, they repeatedly went into the reactor buildings to bring the situation under control. With all power lost, everything had to be done by hand with whatever means they could devise, instead of by remote control.

I knew that many of these people who threw themselves in harm's way had been born and raised locally, in Fukushima. I tried to imagine them struggling on in pitch darkness, stunned and terrified by the critical situation.

Fukushima Daiichi power plant was built on land that, until the end of the Second World War, had been employed as a training site, known as the Iwaki army airfield.

At the time of the disaster, on March eleventh, 2011, I was in the midst of writing the first book in a non-fiction series titled *Last Testament of the Pacific War* (2011, Shōgakkan), about the tragic kamikaze attacks in which so many young people lost their lives.

Coincidentally surrounded by enormous quantities of documents on the war, thanks to my research, I was already aware of the historical significance of the site where the Fukushima plant now stood.

Now, a new tragedy had unfolded, here on the same ground where at the end of the Pacific War, in a situation where there seemed to be no tomorrow, pilots had learned to fly and had practiced their kamikaze attacks. As I imagined these men, in darkness and despair, holed up in their control rooms right next to the reactor buildings, the word that came to mind was 'fate'.

Just as in wartime (though in a sense it was an even crueler situation), men struggled on, refusing to retreat, with no sign of an end. How were they able to endanger their own lives by staying on and even storming repeatedly into that fearful darkness?

They stood on the brink of death.

It was not only the threat of personal death they faced. This Damoclean sword hung over their families, their homes, indeed their very nation. I wondered: *how does one feel and behave in such a situation?*

Their efforts were insufficient to completely prevent radiation damage. At the last minute, though, they managed to avoid the ultimate disaster of widespread contamination from a ruptured containment vessel.

This book does not aim to tackle the pros and cons of nuclear power. It will not even enter into the 'for or against' discussion. An ideological debate on the rights and wrongs of nuclear power would only cloud the human issue of the people who risked their lives.

My only wish is to present the truth about what happened, how the people at the front line felt, and how they coped at the time. My hope is to help people, whether they support or oppose nuclear power, to help them understand what actually happened when that massive earthquake and tsunami struck.

This is the story of the people who fought a heroic battle, who steadfastly maintained their sense of duty and loyalty to their people, holding out to the very end, under the leadership of one man: Masao Yoshida.

Ryūshō Kadota
November 2012

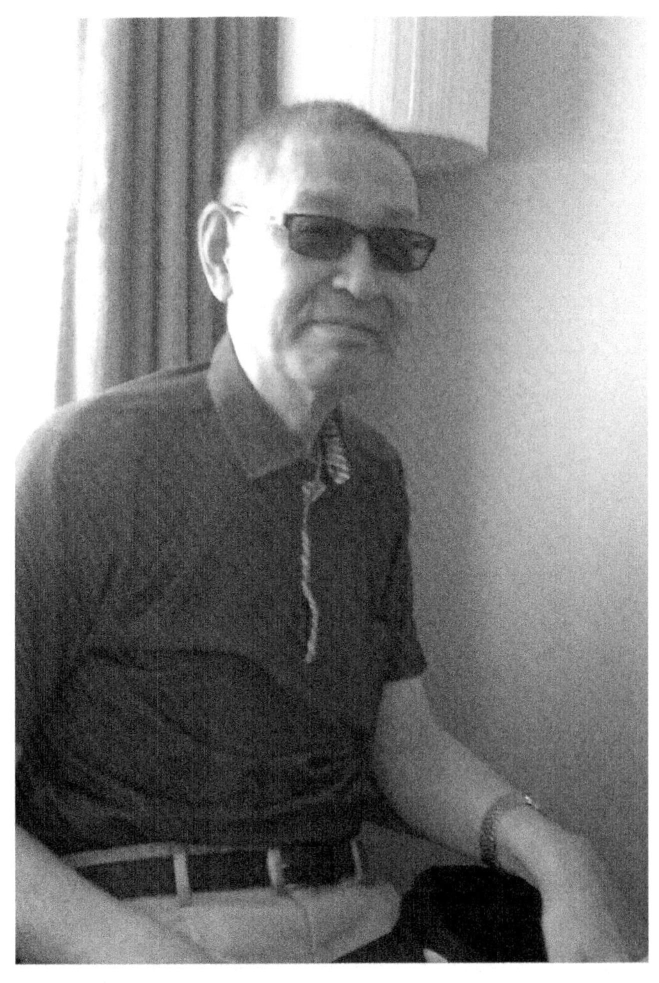

Masao Yoshida during interviews for the book, shortly before collapsing of a brain hemorrhage.

Source: Ryūshō Kadota

Prologue

The boy gazed out to sea.

The waters off Fukushima have a special hue unknown in the tropics; a peculiar deep indigo with a hint of grey. Completely different from the emerald green of tropical seas, on this particular day it reflected the sparkling sunshine of summer, creating a beautiful glittering horizon.

Many who visit the Hamadōri region of Fukushima are charmed by its deep, enchanting sea. This boy, born and raised here, knew no other. For him, this wide, endless indigo Pacific was the very essence of the sea.

The time was the late 1960s; the place, the rural county of Futaba, in Fukushima prefecture.

The army airfield at Iwaki had served as a training field for army pilots during the war, and the ground where the boy stood still retained some of its wartime pavement.

The airfield, which at the end of the war was home to pilots training to fly kamikaze attacks to their own deaths, and the cracked remains of its concrete buildings overlooked the Pacific from the top of a thirty-meter cliff.

There was a meadow at the top of this cliff. In it, a relic of the grim days of the Pacific War, when even mere survival was difficult, stood the lonely derelict ruin. For the local boys, it was an ideal hideout.

Against the background of the boundless ocean, they could play, carefree and without interference from anyone. No adults ever came here. Only a few kilometers from the town, they could cycle out here easily, instantly transforming it into their own exclusive playground.

It was in the late 1960s that they suddenly started to hear the hammering of development.

The boy, born in 1958, the first son of a farmer in the town of Futaba, was named Ikuo Izawa. About half a century later, on March eleventh, 2011, inside the nuclear power station that towered there, destiny was to make him a pivotal figure in the fight to prevent an unprecedented catastrophe.

At the moment that the tsunami triggered the worst nuclear accident in history, Izawa was the shift supervisor in the control room between the Unit 1 and Unit 2 reactors. He was to remain at his post until the end.

But the boy Izawa could not have foreseen the cruel fate that awaited him.

At that time, having reached the upper grades of elementary school, he had recently expanded the scope of his activities. Though previously he had rarely been able to visit the airfield, he had recently started to cycle out there more frequently.

In one sense, this made him a valuable witness to the development and construction of the power plant, from before it even started.

The official history published by the neighboring town of Ōkuma in March 1985 describes the event as follows:

"With the encouragement of the Fukushima prefectural government in attracting a nuclear power plant, and the assistance of TEPCO in choosing a location, an ideal site of almost two square kilometers in Chojahara district was selected and announced on October first, 1960. The smooth progress of the development may be attributed to TEPCO's concerted consensus-building within the local community. During the Second World War, there had been an airfield in the Chojahara district, and the level woods and fields of the coastal terraces were later used as saltpans. Construction of Unit 1 commenced in December 1966, and installation of the reactor vessel was completed in June 1968."

When winter came to Futaba, it used to be normal practice for the breadwinner of each household to head for warmer urban regions to find seasonal work, since there was little to be had amid the ice and snow of northern Japan. The local government's dreams of economically vitalizing the region with a nuclear power plant project were a perfect match for TEPCO's desire to build its first plant in the region, and as a result, construction of Unit 1 at the Fukushima Daiichi Nuclear Power Plant began in 1966. "Daiichi" is the Japanese for "first" or "number one" and "Daini" is "second".

One of those at TEPCO who was particularly keen to have a plant built was the president of the time, Kazutaka Kikawada, who was from Yanagawa, a town in what is now the city of Daté, also within Fukushima prefecture. The poverty of the people of Hamadōri, obliged to become migrant workers every winter just to make ends meet, very likely contributed to his determination to site a power station in the region where he grew up.

It was just at this time that the boy Izawa was making the place his playground. He can never forget the day that a village seemed to have miraculously appeared there.

One day Izawa noticed that dozens of bungalows had been built in clearings in the woods, and that the people who had taken up residence there were not Japanese!

They were people that a country boy would normally never meet: people of all races – they were all *gaijin*. The village was the new home of the General Electric workers who had come to build Unit 1.

The engineers who came to Hamadōri in Fukushima had brought their families with them, so of course there were small children, too. Small parks and community halls were built, and around them tightly-packed rows of bungalows. There was even a small school.

Izawa and the local boys had no idea what these people were there for. It wasn't until much later that they found out that the technicians and their families had come to build the first reactor unit.

Reactor Unit 1 at Fukushima Daiichi was built by General Electric, enabling a technology transfer to Toshiba and Hitachi, followed by the construction of Unit 2 in collaboration with Toshiba, while Units 3 and 4 were built by Toshiba and Hitachi respectively, steadily progressing along the route to purely domestic production.

Izawa and his friends, of course, knew nothing of that and referred to the settlement simply as GE Village. Despite the language barrier, it didn't take long for boys of the same age to make friends. With signs and gestures, playing with the American boys soon became more fun than anything.

He'd often invite his friends, "Hey! Wanna go over to the village, later?"

One attraction was that the American boys had radio-controlled planes, something almost unheard of at the time. In the late sixties, there was probably no other boy in Hamadōri with a radio-controlled plane. For Izawa and his friends, it was irresistible.

Izawa and friends taught the American boys how to play marbles the Japanese way, and their card-throwing games known as *menko*, while the Americans showed them the delights of RC planes.

Together, on an airfield where pilots had once trained for kamikaze attacks, American and Japanese boys amused themselves with RC planes. The Japanese boys were allowed to launch the fifty-to-sixty-centimeter planes into the wind. They would make sure which way the wind was blowing, run into the wind and hurl the planes with all their might. If they got their timing right, the planes would soar up into the sky, but if they failed, they would crash ignominiously to the ground.

The American boys would shower Izawa with abuse when he got it wrong, but the English profanities meant nothing to him. Soon they'd all fall about laughing and Izawa would try to launch the plane again.

Here, looking out over the vast Pacific, this was how they amused themselves.

One of the boys Izawa became particularly friendly with was a boy his own age who had an older brother and a younger sister. Izawa often visited the boy's home.

The boy's blonde mother made him welcome and always treated him to chocolate and fruit juice. One day Izawa received a card. It was an invitation to a Christmas party.

The time and date were written inside and the place was to be the boy's house. Izawa and one of his friends were invited to a real, family Christmas party.

Though over fifty years old now, Izawa remembers it well. Even in those days, more than forty years ago, Christmas was celebrated in Fukushima, but this American Christmas was completely different from the Christmas that Izawa knew.

First, there was the Christmas tree. The boy's father had felled a tree from the surrounding woods and brought it home to decorate. To the schoolboy, Izawa, it seemed to tower over his head. I can't have been a real fir tree as there are few in the region, but the father had managed to find some other similar kind of tree, he recalls.

The next surprise was the mother's homemade Christmas cake. He'd never seen a multi-layered cake like this. In fact, the only "cake" he'd ever had was shortcake, so the memory of stuffing himself on slices of this huge cake – the texture, the flavor – all remain vivid today.

After that, they all sang songs together. It was such fun that the memory of his first ever Christmas party has stayed with him all his life.

However, once Unit 1 was complete, without warning, the Americans all disappeared. Even the GE village itself was suddenly gone. Like a holiday romance, the friendship was over and lived on only in Izawa's memory.

It was from this period, Izawa realized in retrospect, that his father, the farmer, had stopped going away on seasonal work every winter.

Until then, his father had left home at the end of the growing season in November to work somewhere warmer until the snow-cover melted in the following March. But as the project progressed and the power plant was completed, more work became available in supporting industries, and Izawa's father became able to spend winters at home with his family. For Izawa, the construction of the nuclear power plant marked the beginning of many changes.

Now, hardly anyone knows of the existence of GE village. At the end of the 1960s, soil excavated during the lengthy construction of the plant was heaped into a small hill south of the plant. To the north from this hill, later known as the lookout, you could see the full extent of the Fukushima Daiichi nuclear plant site, while to the east lay the indigo horizon of the magnificent Pacific.

There is some historic video footage of the huge tsunami that struck the Fukushima Daiichi plant soon after the earthquake.

That footage, which shows the tsunami soaring irresistibly above the bluff and crashing against the buildings, was shot from this hill. The parking area in the foreground below, to the north of the hill, is where the GE village once stood.

Whenever he went there, Izawa would recall the village and the days of his youth.

Sometimes he looks back with nostalgia at the course he set for himself from then on: graduating from the local technical high school, joining TEPCO and becoming one of the operators in the control room for Units 1 and 2, and ultimately becoming the shift supervisor in charge there.

But he never even dreamed of the unprecedented disaster that would befall the facility on his own watch.

Was it the will of God that led Izawa and his staff to risk their lives in the struggle to preserve their homes and families? Or was it some inescapable destiny that they were born with? Izawa still isn't sure.

Magnitude 9

Out of the blue

Day 1—March 11, 2011 14:30

It was an ordinary Friday afternoon.

Fifty-six-year-old Masao Yoshida, superintendent of the Fukushima Daiichi nuclear power plant, sat alone in his office on the second floor of the main administrative building working on some papers.

Soon, at 15:00, there would be an inter-departmental function – an annual get-together including employees from the Fukushima Daiichi plant who were seconded offsite as well as TEPCO staff at the Fukushima Daiichi plant who worked outside the nuclear section. It was a function which constituted a social event as well as an official one.

Employees who usually worked offsite had come back to Fukushima Daiichi specifically for the event. Yoshida was still busy but, with one eye on the clock, he used the few minutes before the meeting to read through documents and apply his official seal where required.

It was a spacious office. In front of his substantial desk stood a conference table and beyond that the standard coffee table and sofa set.

His seventy square meter room made an entirely appropriate place for entertaining the guests of the head of a plant that could produce a mind-bending 4.69 GWe (gigawatts electrical); it also fulfilled its designed purpose as a highly functional office.

Suddenly, with an unfamiliar rumble, the earth began to shake. It was 14:46 on March 11, 2011.

"It's a quake!" he thought.

Yoshida immediately put down his papers and stood up.

For a nuclear power plant, coping with earthquakes is a grave matter and constitutes just one of the important disaster scenarios that he needed to bear in mind at all times.

TEPCO had already experienced one large earthquake, four years earlier, when the M6.8 Niigata-ken Chūetsu-oki Earthquake of 2007, recorded at 993 gal, shook the Kashiwazaki-Kariwa nuclear power plant on the Japan Sea coast, causing an automatic emergency shutdown of the reactor, known as a scram, and an electrical fire.

At the time, Yoshida had been head of the Nuclear Asset Management Department at TEPCO headquarters, and hence one of the executives responsible for restoring the plant.

On that occasion, an electrical short at the Unit 3 transformers had caused a fire. Because of the earthquake, their fire hydrants were out of order, and they had had to call on the local fire service to control the fire.

"I hope it's nothing serious," he prayed.

He remembers vividly how, despite his entreaty, the shaking got worse. In fact it was so strong that, even holding on to the edge of the desk, he had trouble standing.

The ominous rumbling grew louder and the TV that had stood diagonally in front of his desk crashed to the floor.

The sound of rupturing battered at his ears as the ceiling panels disintegrated and fell to the floor.

The swaying had started as a horizontal motion, but before he knew what was happening, it had changed to a vertical pulsing.

"Oh heck! Must get under the desk, . . ." he thought, but he found he couldn't even crouch down. At more than one hundred eighty cm tall and over eighty kilos he was a well-built man, but it was all he could do just to hang on to the edge of the desk and remain standing until the tremors had run their course.

"It was the strongest quake I'd ever been through," he reminisced. "At that point, I remember thinking that the reactor would scram (i.e. execute an automatic emergency shutdown). It was really long. The swaying must have lasted about five minutes, I'd guess. I just had to hold on to the edge of the desk there and put up with it, alone in the office, until the swaying stopped."

This was a huge earthquake. As soon as it finally ended, he simply flew out of the office.

He had lots to do. First he had to get to his command post, the emergency response center (ERC) in the quakeproof building (QPB) and take control of the situation. Just a week before, on March fourth, they had held a drill to test their response to a severe earthquake, and their earthquake response procedures were something that they refined on a daily basis. If everything went as planned, there should be no problem.

The QPB had been completed only eight months earlier in July 2010, in response to the Niigata-ken Chūetsu-oki Earthquake four years before in 2007.

The new building was constructed on huge rubber dampers to absorb seismic energy. Besides housing the ERC, it was fully equipped for communications, with radiation-proof air-conditioning and its own electrical generators.

If you counted the contractors as well as TEPCO staff, there were more than six thousand people employed at the Fukushima Daiichi plant. Of those, about twenty-four hundred worked within the restricted area containing radioactive materials. Responsibility for all those lives lay in the hands of Masao Yoshida.

Yoshida was concerned only with preserving two things: those six thousand lives and the reactors.

Outside the door of the director's office lay the general affairs department, but when he saw it, Yoshida was lost for words. Just as in his office, the ceiling had collapsed, but here it was even worse - lockers had toppled and papers were littered everywhere. There wasn't a place to put a foot down.

Yoshida's days of hell had started.

Scram

Day 1—March 11 14:46

The reactor building and the service building containing the reactor control rooms, located roughly four hundred meters southeast of the director's office, were hit simultaneously.

"It's a quake!"

"Get down!"

"Hang on!"

At the time of the quake, the shift supervisor in the control room for the Unit 1 and Unit 2 reactors, which was located between the two, was fifty-two-year-old Ikuo Izawa. Just by chance, the usual scheduled shift supervisor had gone to hospital for his regular in-depth medical examination, and Izawa, head of another crew, was substituting for him.

The moment the shaking started, Izawa stood up from his desk.

Operation of the reactor lay in the hands of the shift supervisor and his crew. These technicians, masters of the knowledge and skills required in the operation of nuclear power facilities, worked shifts around the clock. In the hierarchy at TEPCO, all of them belonged to the Operation Management Department of the Fukushima Daiichi plant.

At the Fukushima Daiichi plant, the six reactors were grouped in pairs, Units 1 and 2, 3 and 4, and 5 and 6, so there were three control rooms. Izawa was in charge of the teams responsible for operating Units 1 and 2.

When there is an earthquake, the operators need to check numerous parameters. The control room covers seven hundred square meters. In Izawa's control room, operational control panels filled the walls, with those for Unit 1 on his right and those for Unit 2 on his left. Amid the bedlam of shouts and commands to take cover that rang out as soon as the shaking started, the operators closest to the control panels reflexively grabbed the handrails in front of them.

But this was no ordinary earthquake. With a magnitude of M9.0, it was on a scale that none of them had ever experienced, and it immobilized every one of them. Those who had not managed to grab the handrail at the outset were completely unable to make their way to the console.

Some remained standing, while others rode out the quake sitting on the floor. With his right hand Izawa tried to stop the computer display in front of him from falling to the floor, while with his left he held himself upright by gripping the edge of the desk.

"Don't move! Stay where you are!" he shouted to his crew, but with the incredible shuddering and shaking it seems unlikely that anyone heard him.

The lurching got worse.

"It's going to scram."

"Scram" is the term for the emergency shutdown of a reactor. When a reactor is subjected to the oscillation of an earthquake, or some other abnormal event, the control rods (see diagram page ix) are automatically inserted into the reactor core to shut down the fission reactions. These control rods work by absorbing neutrons and retarding nuclear fission in the core.

If this scram does not occur automatically, a manual shutdown requires a series of steps to insert the rods.

Izawa's warning had reached the other operators, but the violence of the tremor ensured that every one of them had the same thought in mind.

Noboru Homma, the thirty-six-year-old deputy shift supervisor explained: "When Mr Izawa the shift supervisor yelled 'Scram,' we were already thinking the same thing. There are two systems for the scram signal, A and B, and unless both systems send the same signal, we don't get a full scram. When only one system works, we get what we call a half scram, and that's what we actually had at Unit 1 when Mr Izawa shouted."

A little to the rear of the center of the control room, commanding a view over the whole room, stood the shift supervisor's desk and next to it, his deputy's. Homma was sitting in the deputy shift supervisor's seat close to the control panel. The other operators' chairs stood around the central table in front of the shift supervisor's position.

Each crew normally comprised a team of eleven, including the shift supervisor. In addition, there were usually two or three trainees there. The operators were divided, by experience and length of service, into main and assistant operators. On this day there were fourteen people in the Control room of Units 1 and 2.

At that moment, the console showed a half scram.

"Unit 1, half scram!"

As Homma yelled to Izawa, Unit 2 went into half and then full scram.

"Unit 2, scram!"

Next, Unit 1 went into full scram.

"Unit 1, scram!"

"CRs fully inserted," added Homma, referring to the control

rods. The shaking was so violent, he was worried that the service building, in which their control room stood, might itself collapse.

With all the noise from the creaking and groaning of the whole shaking building and alarms sounding from the console, Homma's voice didn't reach Izawa though he was only a few meters away.

"I couldn't hear exactly what Homma was saying. But as he looked at me and yelled, he pointed at the control panel with the lights showing that the reactors had scrammed, so I realized that both reactors had shut down," said Izawa.

The panels at which Homma was pointing displayed vital information. There was a block of red lights in eight columns of seven. The top right lamp was the A-system and the top left the B-system.

When they were red, it meant that the reactor had scrammed. This situation was one of those things the operators had had drummed into their skulls.

To Izawa too, those red lamps confirmed that both reactors had scrammed.

Izawa waved a hand toward Homma, to show he'd understood. The successful scram meant they'd safely passed the first step of the emergency.

"There is a state of mind where we think 'For God's sake, shutdown quickly,' because once the reactors scram properly, things are moving in the right direction."

Once the control rods are inserted into the reactor core, the emergency shutdown is underway and things can move to the next stage. As the tremor continued to shake the control room, Izawa and his crew just had to hope that things went as smoothly as they had done in drills.

To safely secure a nuclear reactor under an emergency situation, the first step is shutdown of the fission reaction, the second is cooling off the reactor and the third is containment of any radioactive leak. Only after these three steps – shutdown, cooling and containment – have been completed, can the reactor be said to be under control.

Izawa and his crew of technicians had to carry out these three steps and bring the reactors under control by dissipating the immense energy accumulated inside the reactor. The proper execution of all three steps was up to them alone, but the first step was now complete.

Eventually the shaking ceased. In the control room, the alarms continued to ring and now, adding to the racket, there was the shrilling of a fire alarm.

That fire alarm was probably set off when sensors detected not smoke, but dust raised by the shock of the earthquake. There was also another alarm, a kind of throbbing noise, indicating abnormal readings on the control panel.

As soon as they were able to move around again, the operators flocked to the console. It was part of the almost instinctive nature of the highly-trained nuclear reactor operators to inspect the console whenever there was anything unusual. As might be expected, the violent shaking of the earthquake had immobilized them, but the moment the motion started to subside, they were at the console reading the figures and other indicators.

What with the noise of the fire alarm, the control panel alarms and the shouts of the operators, the control room was a hubbub, as confused as a battlefield.

Each operator read out the data he was responsible for, while Izawa had to acknowledge each one orally with the word "*Ryōkai!*"

"MSIV, closed!"

"MSIV, closed! *Ryōkai!*" the voices mingled. MSIV was the Main Steam Isolation Valve. The steam that flowed from the reactor to the turbines was the most important element in generating power, and this valve closed the pipe that carried it. Closing it would isolate the reactor from the outside world. If the steam continued to flow to the turbines it was possible that radiation might escape somewhere. To avoid that risk, closing the valve would make sure the reactor was kept in 'quarantine.'

That was when they learned that there was no longer any power from outside the plant. The external electrical grid had failed due to the earthquake.

"Power's down, you know," Homma called to those around him, referring to the usual external grid supply. Overriding his, another voice rang out.

"Start the diesels!"

"Start the diesels! *Ryōkai!*"

The diesel generators were the emergency power supply for use in precisely this situation: when an earthquake or other disaster cut off power from the grid. Whatever the reason for the AC supply to be cut off, these diesel generators were essential to provide power to run the equipment.

The diesels were also crucial to the second step of the process, that of cooling the reactor. In an emergency, they were literally a lifeline. And they started up without incident.

At the same time, Izawa was notified that the Emergency Core Cooling System (ECCS) was ready to be activated.

"ECCS on standby."

"ECCS on standby. *Ryōkai!*"

The operators reported to Homma, their deputy shift supervisor, and he repeated the information to Izawa. Izawa then repeated that back to him and finished off with his own *ryōkai* in acknowledgment. This was to ensure that everyone knew exactly what was going on. Everything was proceeding exactly as it always had done in their regular drills.

"It's all going smoothly," thought Izawa. Everything was being done by the book, or rather, just as they'd done in their drills. At this point none of them even imagined the catastrophe that was about to befall them.

Emergency Response Center

Day 1—March 11 About 14:50

Yoshida ran out of his office on the second floor of the main administration building and down the stairs.

On his way, he found that the fire doors had closed, so he had to take the long way around, through the building, to reach the parking lot at the front. This was the designated assembly point for evacuees in case of earthquake or other disaster.

March in Fukushima is cold. That day's minimum was minus 1.4° Celsius and the maximum only 8.3°C. The staff had all dashed outside just as they were, and hardly anyone was wearing a coat. He saw people with worried faces shivering. Spotting a group of people from the General Affairs section, Yoshida immediately issued instructions.

"Find out if anyone's hurt. Take a roll call for each crew and make sure everyone is accounted for. And find anyone who's missing," he ordered, before hurrying into the quakeproof building beside the parking lot.

As explained earlier, the seismically isolated building, built in response to the lessons learned from the Niigata-ken Chūetsu-oki Earthquake, had been completed only eight months earlier. In the event of a major accident or natural disaster, the staff could hold out there and respond to a variety of situations.

As superintendent of the plant, Yoshida was naturally also responsible for emergency response at Fukushima Daiichi. On the second floor was the emergency response center, which included a room set up for videoconferencing with TEPCO headquarters.

It was a little before three o'clock when Yoshida entered the ERC for what was destined to be a month under siege, working around the clock.

"Have they scrammed?" he asked the members of recovery crew who had started to assemble to the left of the entrance. There were already about thirty people in the room, and more followed Yoshida in.

"It's fine, chief. They've all scrammed properly."

"Good."

Yoshida took the chief's seat at the conference table. The heads of each section were already there – Power, Recovery, Technical – all the essential emergency teams. Everyone looked tense.

"First, make sure we have no fatalities," he said, looking around their faces. "That's the kind of situation we have, so, don't get flustered. We need to go carefully, by the book, verify everything and act accordingly. Don't rush."

The section heads, seeing Yoshida's stern look, nodded to show they understood.

Fukushima Daiichi has six reactors numbered 1 to 6. With all six running together, they could produce 4.69 GWe (gigawatts of electric power) and supply the whole of Tokyo and the metropolitan region.

At the time, Units 1 to 3 were in operation but Units 4 to 6 had been shut down for routine maintenance. This involved shutting down each reactor completely, exchanging the fuel rods, and checking the piping and machinery for wear, damage and leaks. The Electricity Business Act requires such an inspection every twelve months, give or take a month.

Only three reactors, Units 1 to 3, were running when the quake hit.

Responsibility for stabilizing all three reactors and resolving the situation lay firmly on Yoshida's shoulders.

Tsunami

Ten meters of complacence

Day 1—March 11 About 14:50

As the tremors subsided in the control room between Units 1 and 2, someone called Izawa from behind. It was fifty-five-year-old Kikuo Ōtomo, the shift supervisor of the Power Generation section's Work Management group.

The Work Management group was responsible for making arrangements for the tasks required for operating the reactors, carrying out safety checks and other work. Their office was in the same service building, on the right, just down the corridor from Izawa's Unit 1 and 2 control room.

Ōtomo had just run in from there with a dozen of his team. The necessity for this whenever something unusual occurred had been inculcated in these men, who were responsible for the operation and control of the reactors. As they burst in, noises and voices filled the air as the first steps were taken to handle the situation.

"Everything under control?"

"Ah, Ōtomo-*san*! We're just getting under way."

Ōtomo was two years Izawa's senior, hence the "-*san*." The greying shift supervisor was from neighboring Miyagi prefecture. He was unpretentious and earnest, characteristic of people from Japan's Tōhoku (northeast) region, and gave off a particular air of gentleness.

Later, as the situation became more critical, he was to repeatedly risk his life entering the reactor building, but at this point he had never imagined the state of affairs he'd find before him.

Now, immediately after the quake, there were somewhat more

than twenty people in the control room, including those Ōtomo had brought with him.

The shrilling of the fire alarm still rang on, so there was quite a din.

"Somebody, stop that bell!" commanded Izawa. The endless racket was making everyone irritated – something that had to be avoided when calm responses were required.

"*Hai!*" responded one of the operators immediately, and reset the snap-action switch on the wall beside the door of the control room. The piercing noise, which had been ringing since the earthquake, stopped at last.

"With a racket like that going, it's impossible to think straight. I know it's not in the manual, but I felt I just had to tell them to turn it off," Izawa related to me. It was bad enough with the control console alarms going, but at least without the fire alarm they could now hear each other's voices.

Presently, the ERC called to inform them that there was a Major Tsunami Warning in effect. The government's Japan Meteorological Agency had issued the warning and the various media had started to report on it repeatedly.

"Attention! A Major Tsunami Warning has been issued. Whether you are indoors or out, you are advised to evacuate to high ground immediately."

Deputy shift supervisor Homma, on Izawa's order, used the plant's PA system (known as the 'paging system') to relay the message, indoors and out. Homma's voice, amplified by the speakers, echoed around Units 1 and 2.

The reactor building stood ten meters above sea level. The actual electric generation part of the Fukushima Daiichi site stood on bedrock in two large 'steps' cut into the thirty-meter bluff. (See map page x.) The lower, at four meters above sea level, housed emergency seawater pumps and the seawater inlets; while the reactors, turbine buildings and other essential facilities stood on the upper level, ten meters above the sea. Undoubtedly, this ten-meter elevation is what led to the misplaced confidence that the site was invulnerable to a tsunami. Historically, there had never been a tsunami of that magnitude in this part of the world, and no-one took the possibility seriously.

For the personnel at Fukushima Daiichi, the safety of the

ten-meter level was indisputable. But it's when the unimaginable happens that natural disasters occur. That inexorable moment, when they were to learn the danger of underestimating the forces of nature, was approaching.

Izawa, while keeping a sharp watch on the console, had just sent some of his technicians to the turbine building to take care of the procedures required after a scram.

The message broadcast over the PA system urging all staff to take refuge from the tsunami reached them too, but the giant wave was almost upon them.

Close call

Day 1—March 11 About 15:40

"Aaaaagh!"

At that moment, Masamitsu Iga, who was responsible for instructing the assistant operators at Unit 3, saw something he couldn't believe. A muddy, black-brown mass of water was rushing toward him. It was a terrifying sight, like an incensed dragon, swallowing up everything before it.

This was the "major tsunami."

Fifty minutes after the earthquake, he and two of his staff, twenty-three-year-olds Takuya Ara and Takuma Nemoto, were about to check up on the diesel generators in the shared auxiliary facilities building located behind the reactor building. (See map page x.)

They were at the entrance of the building when the tsunami struck.

As mentioned earlier, the diesel generators were an emergency system to provide AC power if, for some reason, power from the grid were lost – an indispensable lifeline if things went wrong.

And the auxiliary facilities building was where the unimagined giant tsunami struck.

Needless to say, the area around the reactor buildings is a high security zone. There are redundant systems for verifying the identity of personnel entering key facilities and denying access to anyone without the proper authorization.

Moreover, the auxiliary services building has two layers of protection, so staff need to be identified twice. First they have their

ID checked at the outer door and enter a small lobby cut off from the world, between two doors. Once the outer door is closed, they must undergo a second ID check before the inner doors will open to allow them inside.

This was where Iga and Ara got into trouble.

The cause of the problem was that when they had left the service building containing the control room, a number of the doors had been open. When the rest of the staff had evacuated the service building during the earthquake the doors had stayed open, and the two of them had simply left the service building and come straight to the auxiliary facilities building. Nemoto, on the other hand, had left through a separate, properly operating door and had officially checked out.

As Iga and Ara had not been properly logged out of the service building, the system considered them to be still inside.

The nuclear power plant's security system had decided that they were intruders, a misunderstanding that was to put their lives in danger.

"When we left the service building, both doors were wide open, so there was no signal sent to the system to say we had exited. The system decided we hadn't left the service building," recounted Iga.

They had each managed to pass the outer doors of the auxiliary facilities building, but when they tried to check in at the inner doors, they wouldn't open.

There are several entrances to the auxiliary facilities building, and now Iga and Ara were each locked in separate rooms. Iga was in a larger room, but Ara's 'cell' next door was tiny.

"Iga-*san*, the door won't open. Is yours OK?" Ara called to his senior in the next room.

"Same here! It won't open," replied Iga. And they couldn't go back outside either.

Ara recalls how astonished he was that neither the inner nor outer doors would open. "Even if we got locked in, there was an intercom which, in normal circumstances, we could use to talk to Security. If they'd only answer the phone, that is. But however often we called, they didn't answer. I guess they must already have evacuated."

And so it was that they were each locked in separate rooms, unable to escape.

"We were stuck and there was nothing we could do to get out. Unless someone outside opened the doors, we couldn't leave. It was one of those situations where you can imagine using a fire extinguisher or something to smash the glass. But the glass was reinforced and it'd be hard to break."

It was just then that Nemoto, who had checked out of the service building, arrived at the building and entered without a hitch.

"What's up? Are you all right?" he asked, calling through the windows after going back outside.

"We can't get through to Security. What's going on?"

At this point, none of them was particularly concerned as they discussed the situation.

"There had been a warning, so we knew about the tsunami, but didn't imagine it concerned us, so we assumed that security just had their hands full with the earthquake and didn't have time to answer the intercom."

Nemoto picked up a nearby fire-extinguisher and asked, "Shall I break the glass from outside?" Iga was still unperturbed and told him to wait a moment.

It must have been three or four minutes later that a totally unexpected sight met Iga's eyes.

He recalls the monstrosity he saw over Nemoto's shoulder.

"It was a dirty, blackish mass of muddy water. Not the usual color of water. It was a mass of brownish black with incredible clouds of spray, and it was bearing down on us."

This wasn't the beautifully hued water of Fukushima's ocean. It was a wild beast that had set its eyes on its prey and was lunging in for the kill.

"Tsunami!" yelled Iga immediately.

"Huh?" thought the nonplussed Nemoto. As he turned to look, Iga screamed at him "Run! Get outta here!" Nemoto turned to the next entry door, hastily logged in and dived inside. Iga and Ara, though, were still trapped in their cells.

With a roar, the tsunami smashed against the building.

The doors held against the initial impact, but water penetrated the seals. It was coming in under the door.

An instant later, the glass in the door where Iga was imprisoned shattered. Whether it was a result of another wave of the tsunami or because a piece of debris had struck the door, Iga didn't know.

As the water surged in, it occurred to Iga for the first time that he might die. The water gushed relentlessly into the small space where he was trapped.

It's all over, he thought.

"I was swallowed up by the water coming in all at once. Even though it was only a small room, I soon lost track of up and down. The water just whooshed in, and it was like being tossed and whirled around inside a washing machine."

Iga was wearing a helmet, but the strap started to strangle him. Still thrashing underwater, he began to choke, so he released the strap.

Trapped in the next room, Ara, too, began to think his end had come.

Because both the door to his room and the window were smaller, they were sturdier than those of the neighboring room, and didn't break. But the water nevertheless poured relentlessly under the door. It had started to pour in even with the first surge of the tsunami.

Now the water level had reached his chest.

His earlier nonchalance was gone.

"Let me out! Let me out!" he yelled into the intercom. "HELP!" he screamed.

I'm going to die, he thought, but for a moment the rising water, which had reached his chest, seemed to pause. He pressed both his hands and his feet against opposite walls of the tiny room and propped himself, bit by bit, higher out of the water.

It was more than two meters to the ceiling. Ara desperately shuffled his hands and feet, bridging up slowly toward it.

But he couldn't keep completely clear of the water. With his feet pressing against the walls underwater, he managed to keep his head and chest above the surface.

Though the flow had slacked off, the water was still slowly rising. There were only forty or fifty centimeters to go. If this carried on, sooner or later he was going to be submerged.

Aaaagh! This is it. I'm finished! he thought.

He was almost ready to give up. It was hard to imagine how he could survive a situation like this. But death had crept up on him under circumstances he had never foreseen.

Images of his family appeared, and disappeared. For the unmarried Ara, this meant his parents, who had brought him up.

"For me to die before my parents was inexcusable. If I were to die, I knew they'd be so sad. I couldn't handle this feeling that I had failed them—"

Thoughts that never normally occurred to him spun around in his head.

"I'd hardly ever felt that my parents were important to me, or anything like that, but at that moment they were the first thing to cross my mind. It kind of reasserted something I'd half forgotten: that parents are something precious."

In the next room, Iga, who was still being swirled around, also recalled his family.

Iga reminisced on that time on the edge. "Tumbled under the water, my mind too was turned upside down. Looking back, I think for a moment I gave up on life. I was being tossed around in the water and had already swallowed quite a bit. I've got a wife and four kids, aged three to fifteen – three boys and a girl – and I could see them there in my head. I've heard that people recall their whole life just before they die, and that was just what happened to me. I remember thinking, *Oh, so this is what it's like to die by drowning.* It seemed to last a long time, but I guess it was really just a few seconds."

There is a clear difference between the high waves of a typhoon and the wave of a tsunami. Typhoon waves are momentary waves that rise and pound down, to be repeated over and over again.

But a tsunami is different. The whole sea itself rises. The first attack alone may seem like the shock of a typhoon wave, but while the wave peaks and breaks, the tsunami is not just an isolated wave; the whole sea itself mounts up behind it. Which is why the sea can ride over anything and everything in its way, swallowing it all up. Once it has ridden over everything, there is nothing to do but wait for it to recede.

Iga and Ara endured that process and miraculously survived the danger. What more can be said but that it was a stroke of fortune surpassing human understanding?

While the two of them endured the torment, the rising of the waters finally stopped. No, it seemed that little by little the water level was falling!

There was no mistake. The waters had started to drain. The

water that had been about to submerse them had begun to return to the sea.

At that very moment, two of their colleagues from reactor Unit 4 had just lost their lives to the tsunami in the basement of the turbine building there. Iga and Ara were above ground, while the two who died were below ground when the tsunami struck and so lost their lives through simple misfortune. The difference was a matter of luck. A tiny difference threw them on separate sides of the line between life and death.

As the water started to slowly subside, Iga tried to escape his cell. The glass in the outer door of the room had been shattered by the tsunami.

It had created a space for him to escape. He struggled through and then realized his hands were covered in blood. He must have cut them on something.

"Iga-*san*! Iga-*san*!"

He could hear Ara calling from the next room. He was still trapped and was yelling desperately for help.

"You're all right. Look out! I'm going to smash the glass!"

Iga grabbed a log floating in the water in front of him. It was a meter long and at least twenty centimeters thick; he dragged it toward the door of the room where Ara remained trapped. There was a small window in the door.

Ara saw Iga coming toward him with the log.

"That looks just right! *Onegai-shimasu!*"

Ara stepped back and turned away from the window to protect his face from the glass.

"Here goes!"

Iga smashed the log against the window but couldn't break it. Compared to the window in the room he'd been in, this one was smaller and tougher.

The window that had withstood the force of the tsunami continued to resist Iga's repeated battering.

They began to get worried. The next wave of the tsunami could come at any moment. If they didn't get out now, they might not be so lucky the second time, they realized.

Eventually the glass broke and Iga thrust the log inside for Ara to use as a step to climb out through the window.

When Ara recalled, "I managed to get through the window

once Iga-*san* had smashed it open for me," Iga took over their account.

"I was so afraid of getting caught by the second wave of the tsunami, and wanted to get out of there as soon as we could, so I really hammered that window. I felt I had to concentrate on one spot or it wouldn't break, so I kept hitting at the same point over and over again. It makes you think of the power it must have taken to smash the window in the room I'd been in. It could have been just the water pressure or perhaps something was thrown against the glass, but whatever it was it must have been really powerful.

Relieved to be on the outside at last, Ara shouted, "*Arigatou gozaimasu!*"

"That was close!" replied Iga. "Now we must get to high ground."

The water was still up to their chests. Even though it had started to recede, the opaque, debris-filled seawater that covered the ten-meter level still impeded them.

Looking for the quickest way to gain height, their gaze fell on a tank for fuel oil about twenty meters away. The dome-roofed tank was pretty tall.

"Over there! That'll do."

Feeling the way with their feet as they waded through the murky chest-deep seawater, the two struggled on.

"The oil tank has a kind of wall around it so that even if oil leaks, it can't escape. The space inside this containment wall was full to the brim with muddy water. The wall is nearly three meters high, but there are steps up the outside. So we ran up them and swam across the couple of meters of murky water and reached the tank. There is a spiral staircase up the outside of the tank, so we went up that. It wasn't until we got to the roof that we finally felt we were safe."

The height of the tank was seven point seven meters.

"As high as this, we should be all right."

At last they were able to breathe a sigh of relief.

Nemoto, who had escaped to the roof of the auxiliary facilities building, spotted them there.

"I was so relieved! The water from the tsunami had flooded inside the building. I'd run up the emergency stairwell to the roof, but I was worried sick about the other two. I couldn't stand still, wondering what to do, because they were in trouble for sure, but downstairs was all under water now, so there was nothing I could do to help them. After a while I spotted them, and watched as they managed to climb up onto the oil tank. I'd been so anxious I just screamed, 'Are you OK? Thank God you made it!' I remember that Iga-*san*'s hands were red with blood so I got some hand-towels that I found up there and threw them across to him, so he could stop the bleeding."

But at this point, none of the three knew of the fatal blow that had been delivered to the plant when the tsunami flooded the emergency generators.

Station blackout

Day 1—March 11 15:37

"The diesels have tripped!" yelled the young operator, as a pall of silence fell over the control room of Units 1 and 2.

"What?"

"Whaddya mean, the diesels have tripped?"

This was an absolutely unimaginable situation. "The DG's have tripped" meant that the emergency diesel generators had cut out. Their last lifeline, the backup generators that were supposed to power the plant if an earthquake were to cut off AC power from the grid, had themselves failed. This meant that they had lost their most critical capacity: There was no longer any way to cool the nuclear reactors.

Before the significance of this ultimate disaster had truly sunk into the consciousness of each of the operators, another unforeseen development occurred right before their eyes.

All across the control panels, the lights started to go out. Irregularly, over the course of half a minute or so, they gradually flickered out.

"Argh, What the? . . . Ehhhh?" For a while the room was filled with incomprehensible gibberish from the uncomprehending operators.

"First, the lighting in the control room suddenly went out all at once, and then the lights on the control panels started flickering out. The room lighting went out all in one go, but the control

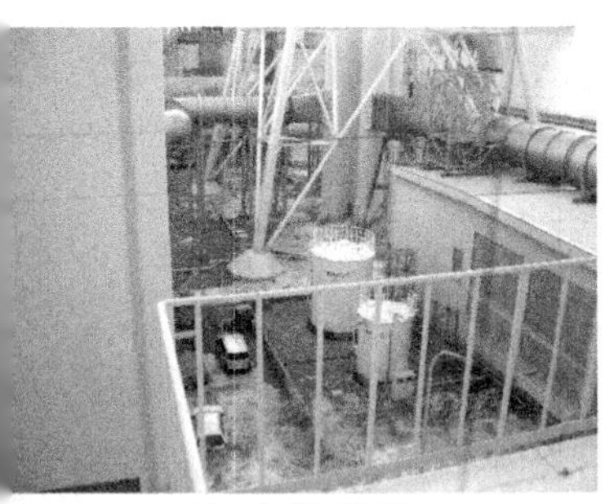

March 11, 15:42

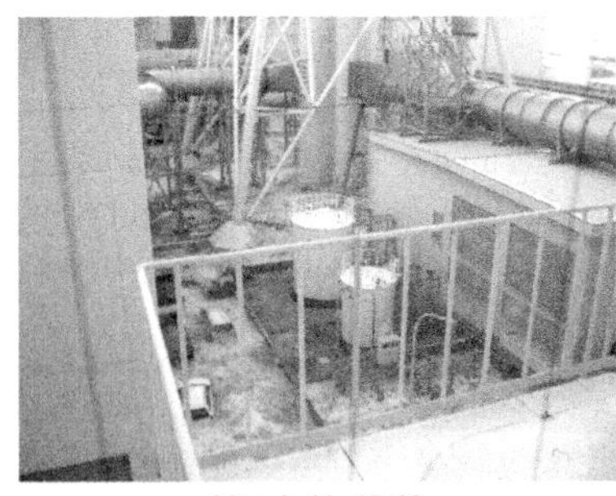

March 11, 15:42

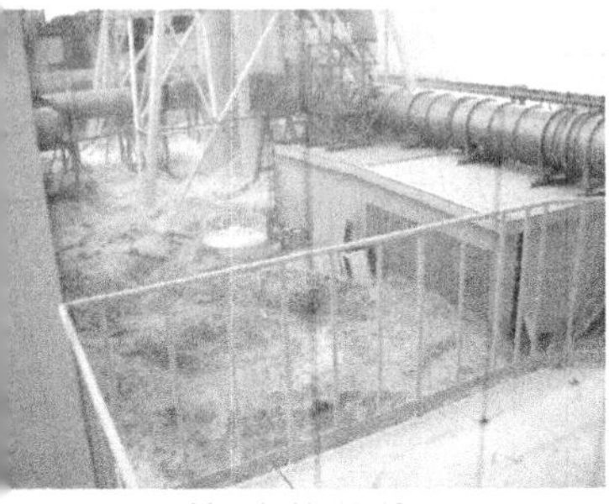

March 11, 15:43

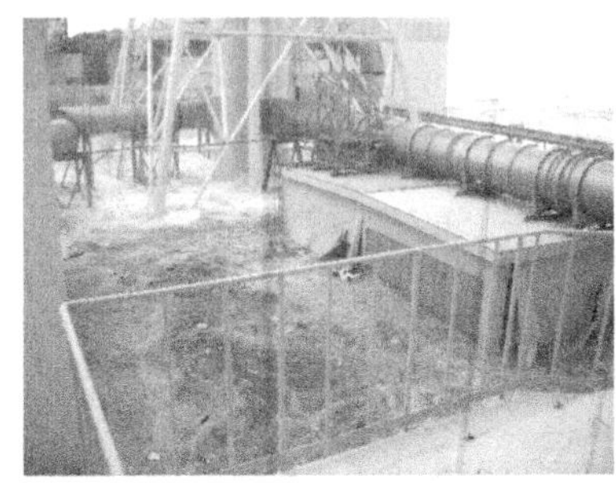

March 11, 15:43

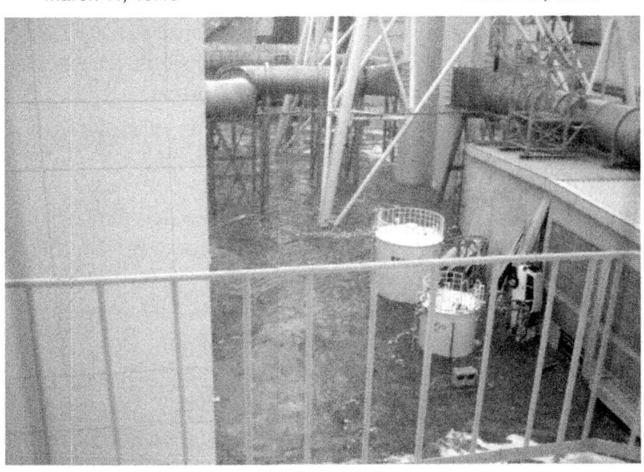

March 11, 15:44

Source: Tokyo Electric Power Co., Inc.

Photos from site ⑭ on page x. Note the white compact car in the lower left of the photograph at 15:42, and in the lower right at 15:44. The water rise can be estimated from the white tank in the center.

panels didn't; they went out bit by bit. Not from the left or from the right; it was nothing like that. There was no order to it; they seemed to just flicker out at random, and all those alarms sounding from each of the control panels died out with them."

Izawa sensed an ominous air, as if some vital spirit had somehow drained from the room.

That deafening fire alarm had already been switched off and the remaining alarms warned of abnormal readings on the panels.

Even that incessant whooping that had gone on uninterrupted since the earthquake almost an hour earlier fell silent as the lights went out.

A hush fell over the control room. In the quiet, the emergency lights on the Unit 1 side of the room glowed faintly. Without them the control room would have been in complete darkness.

"SBO!" shouted Izawa, shattering the silence. 'Station Black Out' meant that they had lost all electrical power, which meant they no longer had the power they needed to keep the reactor cooled.

It was the most desperate situation imaginable.

"SBO!"

"SBO!" repeated the operators, as if testing the reality of the situation, until the room echoed with their voices.

The emergency response center had to be informed of this dire situation. The phone had been off the hook the whole time, and Izawa took it to speak to the operations manager there.

"We have an SBO. The DGs have cut out. This falls under Article 10 of the Nuclear Emergency Act. We are trying to find out what is still usable."

Under the provisions of the "Nuclear Emergency Act," if an emergency specified in the government ordinance occurred, they were required to report it immediately.

For Izawa, the most urgent task now was to find something they could use for power, be it batteries or whatever.

Which generators were still usable? How many batteries still had charge? He had to find out as soon as possible.

Yabai! We're screwed!

That was when it happened.

The door to the control room slammed open as a young operator charged in.

"*Yabai!* We're screwed!" he yelled. As the dumbfounded operators turned toward him he explained: "Seawater! The whole place is full of seawater!" His face was white and he was sopping wet from head to foot.

"Seawater?" retorted Izawa automatically. "Where?"

Now, it was not only Izawa who was asking. Everyone wanted to know where on earth there could be any seawater.

In the windowless control room, Izawa and the rest of the staff had no idea what was going on outside. They couldn't imagine how there could possibly be any seawater. What did he mean?

"Right here. In this building!" answered the dripping operator.

"What?"

It was ridiculous. This was the ten-meter level, which, as its name indicated, was ten meters above sea level. The reactors, the turbine buildings, the service buildings, practically all the important structures, were on the ten-meter level.

Was it even possible for seawater to reach that level? The young operator's ashen face and soaked uniform were sufficient proof that it could, and had.

The reason for the SBO began to make itself clear. From shift supervisor Izawa down to the rank and file, the cause of their astonishing situation began to dawn on them, and it was horrifying!

"After the earthquake, we were busy handling the scram and switching to the reserve power system. After announcing that no one was to be sent into the reactor buildings without the shift supervisor's permission, I had sent a team of operators to inspect them. It was when one of them burst in, soaked to the skin and yelling about seawater that the reason for the SBO clicked," recalled Izawa.

The operator had set off to inspect the reactor, flashlight in hand, and noticing a strange noise had turned back, only to encounter a flood of seawater, he recounted.

This report caused deputy shift supervisor Homma to completely change his perception of the situation.

"Apparently, they had heard an incredible noise while in the reactor building and hurriedly decided to turn back, but there were security barriers between them and the outside where the water was gushing through, and they had had to fight against flow to get out. The report of water pouring into the building was what really brought us to our senses. Realizing that it was a tsunami was what completely cleared my mind."

"Yabai," the word the young operator had yelled, echoed in the minds of the other operators. They were most definitely screwed unless they could find a way to fix the problem, quickly.

Without power, they couldn't even tell what was happening with the Emergency Core Cooling System (ECCS). This was a situation that fell under the trigger conditions of Article 15 of the Nuclear Emergency Act. Izawa had to inform the ERC immediately.

This was how the desperate battle began, in the darkness of the control room, with all power cut off.

The emergency diesel generators and switchboards for the first four nuclear reactors at the Fukushima Daiichi plant were all located in the basements of their respective turbine buildings standing on the ten-meter level. When the plant and its protection were constructed, the predicted height of any possible tsunami had been estimated at only three meters and in 2009, when the predicted height was revised to around six meters, the barriers were strengthened to handle the increased risk.

However there was no protection whatsoever against a tsunami larger than that. Because the diesel generators and their high-voltage switchboards, known as "metal-clad switch gear," had not been moved to higher ground, they were entirely submerged.

It was a prime example of TEPCO's negligence and arrogance toward the power of nature. To put it more strongly, one might suspect TEPCO of brazen self-conceit.

Izawa and his operators, in the darkness of their control room, were quite unaware of conditions on site or of anywhere outside their room.

Outside the control room, the tsunami had left an appalling mess. The ground floor of the service building had been flooded. All the radiation meters and other equipment for use when entering radiation zones had been submerged in seawater, while the racks holding them had been toppled and even carried off by the tsunami.

There was no power, neither AC nor DC. The electrically operated pumps and valves were useless, while the sensors, a vital tool, were wiped out.

And that wasn't all.

Outside the building, it looked just as if the site had been heavily bombed. The tsunami had spread heaps of wreckage, while roadways had subsided, transforming the scene unrecognizably. Mountains of debris denied all access to mere humans.

Meanwhile, aftershocks continued to rock the site. The tsunami warning was still in operation and smaller tsunamis repeatedly battered the seashore.

There could be another big one at any moment. Their situation was desperate.

Grasping the situation

Thinking ahead

Day 1—March 11 15:42

"The emergency power is gone! It's cut out!"

The roar was wrung from deep in his belly and the anguish in his voice instantly sent chills down the backs of the TEPCO employees crammed into the room.

It came from one of the generation crew in the ERC, who'd just received a message from Izawa. The emergency power was out – something impossible had happened.

"Whaddya mean?" spat back Yoshida, the plant manager.

"That's all I know!"

"What's the trouble? Check it out this instant."

"*Hai!*"

That's how Yoshida recalled the exchange with the leader of his power generation crew.

He went on to describe the situation. "I couldn't think what had caused it. I mean, we were being told that the power system that was provided specifically for this situation wasn't working. The only information we had was from the control room, so there were no details to be had. At that point we had no idea how it could have happened. None of us had actually seen the water from the tsunami. All we knew was that it had happened. The generators had started up, had run properly, and then suddenly the power was gone. We could hardly believe it. It was something that just wasn't supposed to happen."

"Up to that point, the TV station had been broadcasting news of the tsunami, but the Meteorological Agency hadn't warned that it was going to be as big as that. I'd imagined that a tsunami might splash the motors for the emergency seawater pumps, which are on the four-meter level. On the other hand, I'd considered that when the trough of the tsunami arrived, the water level might fall below the intake ducts for cooling water, so we'd need to think about what steps to take in *those* circumstances. I'd realized that after a tsunami, we'd need to be starting and stopping all kinds of pumps, and had issued instructions to check the procedures for that kind of thing. But we'd only imagined five or six meters at the most. Nobody had envisaged one of well over ten meters."

It was beginning to make sense at last. It was all because of a tsunami. But this was certainly a situation that no one had foreseen.

"The fact that we'd lost all power, regardless of the reason, meant that we now had to think how to get by without power. This was a completely different scenario from any that we had previously considered."

Yoshida found himself surprisingly composed. His experience of trouble at work had included emergencies both at TEPCO headquarters and at nuclear plants. Somehow he had developed the habit of assuming the worst in an emergency. The possibility that this could end up as badly as Chernobyl had already passed through his mind—which meant that all of eastern Japan was in trouble.

Hmm. This "station blackout" could be the beginning of a worst-case scenario, he thought.

"My mind should have been panicking. But strangely, while part of my mind was concerned that this could turn into another Chernobyl, the other half was telling me to keep calm and start planning. All those things that had to be done started clicking through my brain."

As time went by, information started to flood in.

"All kinds of different data started coming in. News of the tsunami, the fact that the control room was in darkness, the scope of the power cut, the fact that they couldn't read the instruments, all the practical information from the plant. With this wave of information coming in about the actual state of the plant, I was too busy to feel sorry for myself. And I had to process it all and give orders."

He shouted to the recovery crew. "Don't you have any power at all? Then get something running."

They had to get some kind of power source into operation. As long as they had power, the safety system would activate and safely shutdown the reactors. But with power from the external grid gone, and all the emergency generators and batteries out, the only option left was to use generator vehicles. Yoshida sent a request to TEPCO headquarters for generator trucks, and gave instructions to the recovery crew.

"For the moment, work out what you can do," he told them, while his mind turned to the next task.

He had to get hold of some fire engines. If there was no power to cool the reactors normally, then the only way was to cool them directly with water. There was as much water as they could need in the sea; the problem was how to transport it.

"Water was the only way to cool them. But the thing that was continually on my mind from then on was: *What would happen if we couldn't get water in?* I couldn't see any way to do it but with fire engines. There was the distance to worry about. Their hoses might not be long enough to reach from the sea, but they could link the engines in series, I imagined."

Later, many experts were surprised to learn that Yoshida had taken steps to procure fire engines at such an early stage.

"Well, I'd been repairing nuclear plants and operating power plants for a long time, so I'd had my full share of troubleshooting right from when I joined the company. I guess that had all been good training. It's no good begging for something when there isn't any. You have to make do with what you've got. I guess I was resigned to it by then, and had got my second wind. You do what you can at the time, and think about what else can be done, and then you move on to what you're going to need to do it with. That's the way I'd learned to think."

Of the three fire engines stationed at FDI, two had been incapacitated by the tsunami. The only one that was operable was the third, which had, by pure coincidence, been on high ground.

When Yoshida learned of this some time after 17:00, he was already putting in requests for fire engines. This was immediately passed to the Self Defense Forces who soon sent engines to the Fukushima plant, but at this point nobody realized that it was the fire engines that Yoshida had produced that would, by a hair, save the plant from an even greater disaster.

Yoshida was born in Osaka, and bore the well-known hallmarks of people from the Kansai area. He reflected in his colorful Osaka dialect, "We have a saying in Kansai – *Donai-sun'nen?* (roughly: Whaddya gonna do?) I was saying to myself *Come on. Why does this all have to happen on my shift?* There were reports coming in from the reactor all the time, and I had to find a suitable response for each of them. *Donai-sun'nen?* I asked myself repeatedly."

While worrying in the back of his mind that they were in some really deep trouble, he nevertheless managed to devote another level of his mind to devising responses to all manner of lesser problems and giving the necessary orders; in a strange kind of split-level mind.

"I spent that whole day sat in the ERC, video-conferencing and dealing with everything else, without moving from my seat. I don't think I had time for a smoke or a piss all day!" he eloquently recalled.

Rules of procedure

On the other hand Izawa, in the control room of reactors 1 and 2, had gathered all the staff from the service building. The emergency lights on the No.1 reactor side of the room gleamed dimly. The power source for these lights must have escaped the tsunami.

"Listen up!" he announced to the assembled operators immediately after the first tsunami. "We don't know what's going on in the reactors. Before we go and find out I'd like to make sure you carefully follow the rules of operation."

His expression was grim.

"Anyone who goes over there must have my permission and must be back within two hours. Nobody goes alone, only in pairs. No exceptions. If you are not back within two hours we will come and get you. So, even if you don't reach your target, if it looks like it may take you more than two hours, you turn back there and then. And don't forget to write your time of departure and return on the white board as you go out and in." This was how they'd have to operate while there was no way for them to communicate outside the control room. Izawa looked around the roomful of staff, "OK, have you got that?"

"Ryōkai!" came the instant response. "Got it!"

Izawa told me more.

"After the tsunami, the whole power system was down, so even the PA system wasn't working. There was absolutely no way to communicate with the control room while we were inside the reactor building. If we didn't settle on procedures like these, I thought, we wouldn't be able to keep track of people's safety or the progress of operations. It was my call, so I made sure the operators understood right from the start."

These basic rules would be strictly observed throughout the struggle with the reactors that was to follow.

In Izawa's position as shift supervisor, responsibility for the procedures and the lives of the operators was his alone.

"After the earthquake, again after the tsunami, and on many more occasions later, I had to send men into the reactor buildings. Just getting there and back, even without actually doing any work there, would take nearly an hour. If it took a half-hour longer to get there, there wouldn't be enough time left for assessing the situation and getting the job done. By my own reckoning, the longest I could have them actually doing useful work there would be an hour."

Even this was nothing more than an informed guess on Izawa's behalf.

"*A total of two hours,* I told them. At the same time, I insisted that we settle the route to be taken, there and back, beforehand, and once it was decided, there were to be no detours under any circumstances."

An hour after the earthquake, the tsunami had come and gone, leaving the control room for the Fukushima Daiichi plant's reactor units 1 and 2 in a state of emergency, but the basic rules for future operations had been settled.

Outside the plant

At this time, Izawa was not aware that, in response to the earthquake, the off-duty shift supervisors were making their way to his control room.

This was not a requirement in the manual that governed their daily lives, but it was a practically instinctive response for people working in the field of nuclear power to hurry to the plant in the case of an accident to help keep it under control.

One of the off-duty shift supervisors, Katsuaki Hirano, aged fifty-six, had left home after the earthquake and was headed for the Unit 1 and 2 control room.

Hirano had been at home in the town of Futaba, ten kilometers from the plant, at the time of the earthquake. He had taken leave to go to the hospital for a colonoscopy in the morning.

There were five shift crews, A to E, each with its own supervisor, and according to their rotation schedule, it was his turn for duty in the control room that morning.

Hirano was the most senior of the five supervisors and head of the A crew, while Izawa headed the D crew. Because his shift had fallen on the same slot as his previously-scheduled colonoscopy, he'd arranged to swap shifts with Izawa, and after the examination had gone home to rest.

"When the earthquake started it didn't feel like anything out of the ordinary, but the tremors got bigger and bigger until dishes started falling out of the kitchen cabinets and smashing on the floor, so I crossed the verandah that runs around the house and went out into the garden. There are four in our family but my wife, son and daughter were all out at work, so I was alone at home. The shaking felt like a ship in a storm and I couldn't even stay upright, so I knew at once that the reactors would have scrammed. I had to go to the plant right away."

And that day should have been his own shift.

Poor old Izawa! he'd thought.

He couldn't just sit there. Envisaging Izawa, four years his junior, he hurriedly got ready for work. Immediately after the quake, the e-mail on his mobile phone still worked, so he tried to check that his family was safe.

"My daughter was in Tokyo. She said the quake was pretty bad there and asked what she should do. I told her to find somewhere safe nearby for the moment. My wife hadn't replied to my e-mail, so I decided to drop in at where she worked, and set off by car."

But what immediately met Hirano's eyes was the incredible damage from the earthquake.

"The road was covered in bumps, cracks and holes. At the river, the whole road had sunk, so there was now a step up to the bridge which no car could climb. My usual route, the main road, Route 6, was blocked too. It was only four or five kilometers to my wife's workplace, but the traffic signals were all out, because of the power cut, and I wasn't making much progress."

Hirano decided to take a detour, down near the sea, using what local people called the beach road. On the way he found a barrier where it said the road was closed, so he couldn't go any further.

If he had carried on along that road toward the sea, he might well have been caught up in the tsunami, so perhaps luck was with him.

"I did a U-turn and headed back to where I'd started, took the old road past the station in Futaba, and at last reached my wife's workplace. On the way there were telegraph poles leaning at weird angles, fissures in the road and manholes standing high above the asphalt or sunk down into it, and two or three houses had completely collapsed. My wife had already tried to drive home but had failed, she said. I told her the route I'd been able to take and sent her home to take care of the house while I went to work."

At this time, he had no idea of the disastrous situation looming at the plant. Nor was he particularly concerned at what he might find there.

After taking Route 6 again, he eventually arrived at the main gate of the plant at around four thirty, as dusk was falling. It had taken more than an hour from his home.

By then the tsunami had come and gone, but Hirano was totally unaware of that.

"The closer I got to the plant, the traffic heading the other way got heavier and heavier, packing the road with contractors' vehicles from the plant. Mine was the only car going toward the plant."

The exit from the plant was jammed with traffic too, and his was the only vehicle going in. He showed his pass and drove in. (See maps pages viii and x.)

About six hundred meters from the gate, the straight road leads to a crossroads. All he had to do was turn right there and follow the road straight through the cut down to the sea.

The reactor buildings he was aiming for were lined up on the ten-meter level. He headed for his usual parking spot.

That was when he spotted the aberration.

"What the heck? . . ."

As he drove straight down the gentle slope toward the sea, he suddenly found a kind of lake spread in front of him.

A sea of mud covered everything. He couldn't believe his eyes. He was almost taken in by an illusion of the sea risen up onto the land.

He slowed the car, drove past the administration building on the hill and stopped at the edge of the muddy lake. Getting out of the car, he stopped in amazement.

There, blocking the road that was submerged under the lake of mud, stood something huge and round.

"What the? . . . "

He was lost for words. The cylindrical object was an oil tank. There should be two of these enormous tanks down on the wharf, but one of them had been carried up here.

Nine meters tall and twelve in diameter, this tank was a monster that could hold eight hundred tons of heavy fuel oil. It had been washed more than one hundred and fifty meters inland and now blocked the road past turbine building number one.

And that wasn't all.

The tsunami had carried cars and left them, upside down, caught on buildings and pitifully battered. From one of them the horn continued to blare.

There wasn't a soul to be seen, but the horn blared on, making the weird scene before him even creepier.

The thing that surprised Hirano most was the fishing boat.

There it stood, in front of the displaced oil tank. It wasn't technically a fishing boat, but a utility boat that belonged to TEPCO and was used for surveying and radiation sampling at sea. *Whatever.* The only thing that could bring a ship that ought to be floating on the sea to a place like this was at last clear to Hirano.

A tsunami!

The plant must have been wrecked. Only an unimaginable tsunami could have done this. The reality at last began to sink in.

I must get to the control room as quick as I can.

To get where he was going he had to cross this lake of mud. Bracing himself, he stepped in.

At the time Hirano was wearing a black down jacket with cotton pants and sneakers.

"What was it? Only ten to fifteen centimeters of water, I guess. If I'd been wearing rubber boots, it'd have been no problem, but with sneakers the water came right in. I splashed along and just before the tank I found this great big fish, dead, with its white belly up. I've no idea what kind of fish it was, but it must have been about thirty centimeters long."

The scene he was familiar with had been transformed into something unimaginable. Before him lay wood and metal, fences and tiles, all swept into piles of smashed rubbish. He couldn't help but appreciate the gravity of the situation.

"I realized that the puddle of water I was walking through had been left by a tsunami. But it was one heck of a puddle, covering practically the whole of the ten-meter level. At this stage I didn't realize that the power had been wiped out, but it was clear that the pumps down on the four-meter level that were used for cooling the reactors must have been damaged. They'd have been flooded and were probably useless now."

For a nuclear power station, this was a critical situation.

This is going to be a long fight, he thought to himself.

Helpless

When he eventually reached the service building and climbed the stairs to the blacked out control room, he went and stood behind Izawa, who was rushed off his feet, and spoke.

"Hi! How's it going?"

Izawa turned and saw him, and burst out, "Hirano-*san*! You made it!"

Hirano was of medium height and chubby, with greying hair – the epitome of a mild middle-aged man – and there he stood before Izawa.

For Izawa, who thought he had a hopeless battle on his hands, it felt as if a million reinforcements had just arrived.

"It was quite a surprise. I was standing there at the control panel, checking things out, when from behind me came a voice. I turned around and there was Hirano. I was so glad to see him I just yelled out his name. The emergency lights were still glowing dimly on the Unit 1 side, but otherwise it was completely dark. And Hirano had taken the trouble to come. I was delighted."

Izawa had only taken the shift so that Hirano could have his scheduled colonoscopy exam, so Hirano felt he really owed him, which had made him all the more determined to get to the plant. And here he was.

Later, the other off-duty shift supervisors managed to make their separate ways to the control room, but Hirano was there immediately. However, the seriousness of the situation soon turned his agreeable look into a grim one.

"What's the situation?" asked Hirano.

Turning to the panel, Izawa replied, "Er, well, there's nothing we can do!"

"Are you serious? . . . "

For a veteran nuclear reactor operator like senior shift supervisor Hirano, the significance of the situation was obvious. None of the instruments in front of them displayed any information whatsoever.

"The scram was successful and the DGs started up properly. Everything went smoothly until suddenly we lost all power," explained Izawa.

Hirano already knew the situation outside. He had seen the washed-up oil tank and the utility boat out there. It was easy for him to imagine how the power had suddenly been cut off.

"We don't know what state the isolation condenser on Unit 1 is in. We can't tell the water level in the reactors, or the pressures, or anything!"

The situation Izawa described was completely hopeless. His "*There's nothing we can do!*" was no exaggeration at all.

This isolation condenser, located at the top of the reactor building, can cool the reactor by gravity feed for a while even without electrical power.

This kind of cooling device is found only on "first generation" Boiling Water Reactors (BWR) – one of two types of the so-called "light water" type. Fukushima Daiichi, as explained earlier, was built by General Electric and completed in 1971, and so was equipped with this type of isolation condenser.

And the current state of the isolation condenser was unknown.

There are four valves that are used to control the flow of water in the condenser, but the power sources used to open and close them and to monitor their positions, both the AC power grid and the DC battery supply, had been lost.

The cause of the loss of power was flooding by the tsunami, and because the flooding and the consequent loss of power had been gradual, they didn't know whether the valves were open, or closed. They might even be somewhere in-between.

Hirano realized things were even worse than he'd imagined.

Without the control panel to refer to, Izawa realized that, despite the continuing aftershocks and the risk of another tsunami, he was going to have to send someone into the reactor building.

Yoshida in the ERC was in a similar situation and had no data on the isolation condenser. If, hypothetically speaking, it wasn't functioning, then cooling – injecting water – was more urgent than ever.

In due course, the conclusions of the various investigations of the accident and reports in the media circulated the idea that if the isolation condenser had functioned properly, the disaster could have been avoided.

Sixteen months after the accident, in July 2012, Yoshida explained it to me like this:

"My staff were like blindfolded pilots in the cockpit of a plane with its hydraulics and everything else shot to pieces. How were they supposed to get down safely? We'd no way of knowing what position the valves were in when the power went down. The only thing we knew for certain was that we had to stick some water in there fast and keep the thing cooled. So while on one hand we worked out ways to restore power to the plant, we never stopped working on the other side."

Though they each had their own battle to fight, they were all aimed straight at the same target.

Incursion

Pipeline

Day 1—March 11 16:40

Moving to the Unit 2 side of the control room, Izawa explained the situation to Hirano. "Right up until the tsunami, the RCIC (Reactor Core Isolation Cooling) system on Unit 2 was running, but we've no idea what it's up to now. With the power out there's no way to tell."

If there was one thing Hirano was sure of it was that they had to get some water in there. But there was no power to run the cooling system; if there was no power source available at all, that meant the only way left was to find a way to inject some water using the pumps from the firefighting system which didn't rely on an electrical power source.

"It was the only thing I could think of. But, to use the fire pumps to inject water into the reactor, first we had to construct a supply line. The first thing that came to mind was to supply the pumps from the water mains. We talked about getting the mains valves opened; otherwise it wouldn't work. But soon after that we realized that the AM (Accident Management) system had its own fire hydrant network and planned to access it by the evening.

First, we had to make sure the system's pumps were in good order. I sent word to Izawa, that without electric power, this was the only way we had to inject water, so how about it?"

But the experts had already thought of that. At this point, Izawa had already started to set up a pipeline using the water supply that Hirano was considering.

At 4:55 pm, an hour and a quarter after the tsunami had struck, the first squad set off to the reactor building to ascertain the conditions inside. They hadn't yet put on their radiation proof masks. But before entering the building they turned back.

"Everything was still soaked from the tsunami and we didn't have the right kind of radiation meters for those conditions. We made do with some Geiger-Müller tube detectors. The entrance to the reactor building has double doors, so it's completely cut off from the outside. You have to open the outer door, go inside and close it completely before the inner door will open. But as soon as we reached the outer door, the meters were already off the scale," one of the party explained.

It was possible that there had already been a radiation leak inside the reactor building. This had to be reported right away, so they returned to the service building to see what action needed to be taken.

Any operation had to allow for the possibility of a further tsunami. One precaution was to station a junior operator on the roof of the service building to keep an eye on the sea. If there were another big tsunami, first the water level would suddenly drop. A lookout had been posted and if a drop in water level were spotted, they were to turn back immediately. But before any change was noticed, they had detected radiation and had had to abandon the first incursion.

At 17:19 a second squad set out. This time the group included Hirano himself.

"Yes, I went myself. I'd already changed out of my civvies and into the blue one-piece coverall we call a B-suit. At this stage, we weren't using the Tyvek suits that prevent radioactive material from directly touching the skin. There were three of us in the team."

This operation was to have a decisive effect on the water injection operations that were to follow. Hirano and his two colleagues took the stairs down from the control room and headed for the basement. Between the reactor building and turbine building there is a corridor about four meters wide and fifty long, that the operators had nicknamed 'The Pine Corridor' and in the level below a similar one known as 'The Bamboo Corridor.'[1]

1 Pine, bamboo and plum, "Shō, chiku, bai" indicate three descending levels of quality in a variety of goods and services in Japan.

The name was applied because the length and width resemble those of a famous corridor in historic Edo Castle where Asano Naganori, daimyō of the Akō domain in the province of Banshū, precipitated the events which led to the well-known story of "The Forty-seven Rōnin."

Just before the 'Pine Corridor', they entered the basement, where Hirano noticed another dead fish, even bigger than the one he'd seen earlier.

"This one must have been fifty centimeters. I think it was a sea bass. Just the one. Belly up and dead."

The dead fish emphasized the abnormality of the situation here, indoors, in the dark, radiation-control area. The three of them passed it in silence on their way down the stairs. There were still puddles of murky water left from the tsunami, as well as mud, sand and other debris.

In complete darkness, they were dependent on their flashlights. Nobody mentioned it, but they were all aware that another tsunami could come at any moment. They'd be lying if they said they weren't afraid.

"Our cellphones weren't working, so if the lookout noticed the sea level suddenly dropping, someone was supposed to run down and tell us. And we'd already found pools of water all over the basement levels from the first tsunami."

At last the three reached the fire pump room. It was about five meters square. The engines and pumps stood on concrete mountings and beside each was an electric starter motor with its own battery. No external power was required.

"We went inside and switched on the engines from the control board. Once we'd confirmed that they worked, we switched them off again. Leaving them running would be a waste of fuel, and the pipeline to the reactor wasn't ready either, so for the time being we turned them off. We knew they'd work, so we could switch them on again when the pipeline was set up."

The work in the pump room was completed in about thirty minutes. By the time they returned to the control room it was almost 18:00.

Into the lion's den

Day 1—March 11 18:00

Soon after Hirano and his team got back, they started work on the pipeline. By 18:30 they had started to assemble the line that would pour water into the reactor.

With this total power blackout, a task that would normally be done with the flip of a switch in the control room had to be carried out manually. The team was led by Ōtomo, Hirano and his experienced assistant shift supervisor, Katsumi Katō (aged forty-six).

"There were five of us, and about five valves that we needed to open by hand. We were already in Tyvek suits with the full-face masks used when high radiation exposure was anticipated. I didn't think the radiation levels were actually very high yet, but we thought it best to be on the safe side," Hirano explained.

Later, after about 23:00, radiation levels rose and Superintendent Yoshida prohibited further entry to the reactor building. Later on, much was to hinge on this 'lifeline' water supply that they were now working on.

Conversely, if they hadn't built this pipeline, there would have been no way to cool the reactor with water, nor any other way to bring the reactor under control. There is no doubt that these veterans' prompt decisions and swift action at this point were vital in the subsequent efforts to control the plant.

A nuclear reactor expert later explained, "From the accident management perspective, the first people to realize the need to set up this pipeline were the people there on site."

"This pipeline was to be linked to the reactor's emergency core cooling system injection line (the LPCI or Low Pressure Coolant Injection). Surrounding the metal liner to the containment vessel is a wall of concrete about two meters thick with a number of pipes running through it. The point was that the reactor core was inside, and they were constructing a pipeline from the fire pumps to be connected to these, to supply water to cool the reactor."

The pipeline was not devised according to instructions from the emergency response center, but on the initiative of the control room staff. It was the outcome of brainstorming among the veterans in charge there, such as Ōtomo, Hirano and the shift supervisor, Izawa.

Assistant shift supervisor, Katō recalls when Ōtomo brought him the plans showing the layout of the pipeline and its valves. "I remember Ōtomo-*san* saying that, whatever it took, we simply had to carry it out as soon as possible. Then he showed me the plans, which I believe he'd worked out with the other supervisors. Once I'd had a look at them, I was convinced he was right."

All the instructions were laid out, with locations and details of each of the valves that had to be opened. This was the first of many operations in what was later to be called 'the danger zone.'

Shift supervisor Izawa announced that he would go himself, but Ōtomo retorted, "Izawa, you need to stay in command here. I'll go," which was followed immediately by a volley of "I'll go," and "Me, too!" from Katō and Hirano. And that was how the crucial decision on the membership of the first team was settled. Izawa was the shift supervisor, who was forbidden from carrying out work on-site himself and had to stay in command. Katō was the assistant shift supervisor. This was technical site work and, in Katō's mind, he was responsible for leading the work crew. If anyone was to lead the group, it had to be him, he thought.

Thirty minutes earlier, the radiation had already been high enough to send the Geiger-counter off the scale. This meant they would be groping around with no idea whether any water was actually being delivered to cool the reactor at all. The fear must have been considerable. Undoubtedly, each of them had his own thoughts on the selection of the team.

Hirano told me of his state of mind.

"At the time, in Unit 1, and Unit 2 for that matter, we had no idea whether any water was reaching the reactor vessel, so a meltdown could have occurred right while we were working in there. To be honest, it was scary."

It would later be known that at around 19:00 the fuel rods in Unit 1 had started to disintegrate. Though the operators couldn't know the precise situation, they were aware that radiation levels were gradually rising. In the darkness, they searched out the valves and read out their numbers.

Ōtomo added, "Because of the radiation levels, it was best that we seniors went in and left the youngsters behind. Once we'd made sure we knew where to find the valves on our checklist, we got on our way."

Normally, air-conditioners and other equipment running would make quite a bit of background noise, but with the power out it was not only completely dark but also completely silent. Everything was wrapped in a foreboding hush.

With flashlights in hand, the team plodded on until eventually the reactor building loomed in front of them.

"The only thing we had in mind was reaching our target, so we hardly noticed anything else," Ōtomo recalled. Deputy chief Katō, who was with him, added, "When we entered the building, we opened and closed the two sets of doors. These have a bar handle – a metal rod with a black grip at the end. This bar has to be lifted from the horizontal to the vertical, and when you do so it makes a loud *clunk*. Hearing that really made us realize we were committed. That *clunk* reminded us we had a job to do and gave us the push to get on with it."

Once inside the double doors, they were on the first floor of the sixty-meter-high reactor building.

Before them stood the containment vessel, thirty-two meters high and eighteen wide. In the silent gloom, the containment vessel seemed like a wall hanging over them. (See diagram page ix.)

"The containment vessel has concrete walls, but we were there to open some valves, so we didn't have time to waste looking at or worrying about what was behind that looming wall. We were too occupied with the layout of the equipment on the outside of the wall."

On the right, as they entered through the double doors, was a flight of stairs which they silently descended. There were two valves at the first location. One was operated after climbing onto a platform, the other at arm's length in an uncomfortable position.

If the power had been running, this could all have been operated from the control room at the touch of a button. Instead, it had been necessary for these operators to enter the reactor building and do it by hand.

It was a fight against time, and also against the fear of radiation.

"Of course the radiation was on our minds when we went through the doors. I don't know if it was resignation or courage, but once we were inside we knew we simply had to get on with it," Ōtomo told me. Katō explained, "On the panels in the control room there are valve opening indicators with a scale from zero to a hundred percent. These allow us to check how far open the valves really are. But it was all being done manually this time, so we had to take off the protective covers and visually check them one by one. The handwheels were really stiff and each valve seemed to be of a different kind or have different sized pipes. The handwheels on the first ones were about the size of a human face, I guess."

Before moving each valve they had to check the number on it to make sure they were opening the right one, and also to make sure they rotated the wheel the right way.

"Valve 365!"

"Valve 365, *ryōkai!*"

They were both wearing full-face masks, and unless they shouted they couldn't hear each other, so they ended up yelling at each other at the top of their voices.

At the side of each valve was a latch-lever to switch from automatic to manual operation. Once they'd matched the cogs they would start to turn the handle with both hands.

"Twenty-five A, open!"

"Twenty-five A, open, *ryōkai!*"

One by one, they worked down the list. It was not just a race against time but had to be done precisely too.

"We were carrying portable Geiger counters, but what with flashlights in our hands and the need to use both hands on the valves, we'd switched them off. Instead, we relied on our Alarm Personal Dosimeters (APD) to warn us, and I remember listening carefully for the alarm as I worked."

The size of the valves gradually increased, and at the second location, the third, the fourth, their anxiety rose too. But considering that they were moving closer and closer to the core itself, that was hardly surprising.

The last two valves, in the emergency cooling system for the core, known as the corespray system, were located separately on the second floor. One was almost three meters from the floor, and had to be reached by climbing a metal ladder enclosed in a narrow cage.

The valve itself was huge. The wheel was sixty centimeters across. First they climbed to the second floor and then a few meters further, up the ladder to the valve on the outside of the containment vessel.

It took two of them to turn this wheel. Sweat dripped inside their masks and pooled in their eyepieces until they wanted to rip off their masks for relief.

By the time they'd opened the last valve it was almost 20:00–more than an hour since they'd left the control room. This operation was later to become crucially important.

About an hour later, the fuel rods in Unit 1 began to melt and the radiation levels shot up. At 23:00 they were too high for anyone to enter the reactor building and it was declared off-limits.

They had successfully managed to set up a pipeline and secure a water supply, all while it was still possible to enter the building.

None of the water that was subsequently injected into the reactor would have got there without this pipeline. And without it there would have been no way to cool the reactor.

"Of course we were aware of the danger, but somebody had to do it. As operators, it was our responsibility, so it was the natural thing to do."

Even now, Hirano is quite sure: it was, without a doubt, the operators' fierce sense of duty that drove them.

Evacuation

A village elder

Day 1—March 11 About 15:40

Above the unbelievable noise – something out of this world that made his hair stand on end – the elderly man heard a yell from his high-school-aged grandson.

"Tsunami!"

Tsunami? Seventy-nine-year-old former mayor of the town of Ōkuma, Shūrō Shiga, and his wife Tsuneko couldn't believe their ears.

The Shigas' house stood fifteen meters above sea level. It was only three hundred meters from the sea, but there were several embankments in-between and, as it stood so far above the sea, they had never before had any concern about a tsunami.

Located but a few hundred meters south of the Fukushima Daiichi plant, the Shigas were definitely the nearest household to the nuclear plant. The enormous tsunami that dealt a fatal blow to the plant also snapped its jaws at its neighbors, the Shiga family.

The spine-chilling roar, like nothing he had ever heard before, and his grandson's shout of "Tsunami!" reached Shiga's ears just as he was about to get into his daughter-in-law's car in order to evacuate after the earthquake.

The car lunged forward, and Tsuneko glanced back as a staggering sight caught her eye. Above the line of pine trees to the seaward side of the house, loomed a huge black wave, heading right for them.

"Don't stop!"

Their daughter-in-law kept her foot on the pedal and, though the water approached within thirty meters of the car, managed to outrun the tsunami. The emergency evacuation broadcast had probably mentioned the possibility of a tsunami, but they were the Shiga family who lived fifteen meters above sea level. Surely it couldn't have anything to do with them.

They hadn't imagined there might be a real need to evacuate.

"Even if there was a tsunami, there was no way it could reach our house. Well, that's what we'd always thought," Shiga recalled.

"Earlier in the day, my daughter-in-law and her son had driven into town, but had been so unnerved by the earthquake that they had come back. And that was when the tsunami arrived."

The two had come back because of the earthquake. That turn of fate was all that had saved the old couple. And only by the skin of their teeth.

Sad to say, two people in the next house lost their lives in the tsunami, while the house next to that was completely washed away. Even in the Shiga's house, the seawater reached one meter thirty centimeters up the walls.

If the old couple had been alone in the house, they might not have escaped.

Shūrō Shiga was born in October 1931, at Ottozawa in the former village of Kumamachi (now part of the town of Ōkuma) in Futaba county, Fukushima prefecture. There was probably no-one who knew as well as he the transformations that the site of the Fukushima Daiichi plant had undergone.

He had known it when Ottozawa was still out in the wilds. He'd seen it become an army airfield during the war, and then after the war he'd seen the land used for salt pans. He was not merely a living witness to its transfiguration into the cluster of modern buildings that made up the Fukushima Daiichi nuclear power plant, but was also one of the characters involved.

His wife, Tsuneko, who had lived there ever since they married in 1954, recalls, "That noise! I'd never heard anything like it. That awful ripping sound, like something being torn apart. We were all just getting into the car. I was just coming out of the house and looked around, and there it was. A tsunami! Really high, it was. The trees over there, you couldn't see them, the water was so high. Blackish-brown muddy water. Terrible, it was. I couldn't say a word. The next-door-neighbors died, you know. And the house beyond that, the people weren't killed or anything, but the whole house was gone. Washed clean away, it was. If the car hadn't started, we'd have been done for."

If the car had stalled, the Shiga family might well have become casualties. Their daughter-in-law had saved their lives by keeping her foot hard on the accelerator.

More than thirty years earlier, Shiga had suffered damage to his optic nerves during a medical procedure, and, since developing cataracts a few years ago, had gone almost completely blind. Even if you stood right in front of him, he would sense no more than an outline, so he could not visually recognize people.

Which is why Shiga didn't see the tsunami himself. On leaving his home, he was saved the horrific sight of the tsunami, but also missed a last view of his cherished home.

It will be a very long time before any member of the Shiga family is able to return to that house only a few hundred meters from the grounds of the Fukushima Daiichi nuclear power plant. For the Shiga family, living as refugees in Iwaki, their desperate escape has turned into an interminable separation from their beloved home.

The Shigas were a long-established family and their ancestral home was protected by a sturdy earthen wall. According to Shiga's daughter-in-law, this boundary wall reduced the impact of the tsunami.

"The tsunami seems to have stopped at the boundary. It's an old-fashioned earthen wall, a bit higher than most, and it did a good job holding back the water. The gateway was ripped out, posts and all, though. And the water came up more than a meter above the floor, but the Buddhist altar is in a high place so the ancestors' *ihai* (memorial tablets) were safe. I'd shut the door on my way out, so the glass was smashed in, but nothing was washed away."

Just before they were ordered to evacuate again, this time to avoid the radiation spill, Shiga's younger son went back to inspect the damage and found fish washed up in the garden.

"My second boy took my grandson to have a look at the house, and they found this great big mullet, nearly half a meter long, just lying in the garden. I guess it must have ridden up on the tsunami. I asked him why he didn't bring it back!"

Shiga and his wife spent that night at their grandchildren's home in the same village of Ōkuma.

"There was no electricity or water. We had nothing to eat all night. Then, in the morning, there was this announcement. Something about everyone in the ten-kilometer zone had to evacuate, they said. There was a group of people from the town hall walking around telling everybody it was too dangerous here and we had to assemble at the town hall. They weren't using those electric megaphones, you know. It was just staff from the town hall or perhaps it was the fire service, walking house to house to tell everyone. There was quite a racket outside, so we wondered what was going on. Then there was another announcement. There'd been an Evacuation Order. They were sending buses to pick us all up, so we had to assemble at the town hall. When the people heard that, they all swarmed off into town, so we thought we'd better go and see what's up, and headed into town after them."

Thus, on the morning of March 12, following their instructions, the people of Ōkuma assembled at three locations: the town hall, the junior high school and the sports center. The Shigas made for the town hall.

Shiga described how they were unable to get on a bus.

"There were about eight buses, but there wasn't room for all of us. We'd been waiting about two hours at the town hall. It was freezing. Then one of my staff from the old days when I worked there comes along, so I says to him 'We can't hang around in the freezing cold like this any longer. We're going to evacuate in my son's car,' and he says 'You can't do that!' Well, that was what they'd all been told at the beginning, I suppose. But he decided to go and see about it. Went to some 'HQ' or something and asked them what to do, and when he came back he said it was OK now."

As Shiga's son drove off in the family station wagon, with seven or eight people crammed in, one of the younger staff from Ōkuma town hall called out, "Have a safe trip!"

It was already past 10:00 in the morning.

Leaving their precious ancestors' memorial tablets behind, and with nothing but the clothes they stood in, they had no idea how long they were going to be away.

"At that point, we were only told we had to leave the ten-kilometer zone, so, as we had to leave anyway, I said 'Let's go over to my brother's place in Katsurao,' and that's what we did. What was it? Two nights and a day, we stayed there? And then, bit by bit, the evacuation area started growing. Katsurao fell inside the thirty-kilometer zone. That's why we had to evacuate from there, too."

Being almost blind, life in the gym would have been a huge burden for Shiga, so for more than three months he stayed with his daughters in Kawasaki and Yokohama (near Tokyo), and by the time he was eventually settled in an apartment in Iwaki it was already the end of June.

In October 2011, living in a rented room, he reached his eightieth birthday. Since being driven from his ancestral home by the tsunami he hadn't once been back. Though he had escaped with his life, if only just, the *ihai* of his parents and ancestors remained back in the house. Of course, he had not been able to visit their graves in the graveyards near the house at the customary times either.

In August, five months after the disaster, his wife was allowed to make a short visit to the house, but even indoors their radiation meter read a high 46μSv/h, so she wasn't allowed to bring anything back.

"I left the ancestors to guard the house."

Shiga believed the tablets of his ancestors would protect his house. The same August, still at their temporary accommodation, they had had the head priest of the family temple conduct the traditional services for the thirty-third anniversary of the death of his father, though in the absence of his father's *ihai* tablet.

"I was born and raised there. I've got every little corner of the town, especially down by the sea, all packed away up here in my head. Ours is such an old family, we've got two graveyards, only a few minutes from the house. If only the government would put their backs into it and clean it all up so we can go home. You can imagine how the whole area has changed since the power station was built. There wasn't much work in Ōkuma before, but then things looked up. All that kind of stuff keeps coming back to me."

It's no wonder he feels so aggrieved at the tsunami that changed everything, and at the contamination caused the nuclear disaster.

"There was a fellow in charge at the plant called Yoshida. I heard it myself from one of the TEPCO people, that the staff at the plant wouldn't have done all that they did if it hadn't been for that Yoshida fellow. But, if I'd been in his place, and I'd been in charge, I'd have gone into the reactor building and done what had to be done, I reckon. We're both locals. We'd want to protect our home ground."

When leaving his house, the almost blind Shiga hadn't had the chance to savor a last glimpse of his home and neighborhood, nor will he be able to see it if he ever returns there. But he is determined that one day he will return.

Gravely, the eighty-year old Shiga declared: "I'm going back, even if it takes years. TEPCO and the government have simply got to make it happen."

The journalist

Day 1—March 11 14:40

To the south of Shiga's home town of Ōkuma lies the town of Tomioka, about ten kilometers from the Fukushima Daiichi (Number 1) plant.

The southern part of Tomioka is home to another nuclear plant, the Fukushima Daini (Number 2) power station, so the town center is sandwiched between the two nuclear plants. (See map page vii.)

Like those of Ōkuma, the residents of Tomioka, too, were all forced to evacuate.

On the afternoon of March 11, 2011, forty-two-year-old Makoto Kamino, head of the Tomioka branch of the *Fukushima Minpō*, the largest local newspaper in Fukushima prefecture, had finished cleaning out his office and was headed to the local incinerator with ten bags of garbage crammed into his car. A week earlier he'd been told he was being transferred to the head office, and had been getting ready for the move.

With the trunk and all the passenger seats in his beloved 1500 Nissan Tiida stuffed to the brim, he had just arrived outside the office at the entrance to the incineration plant.

That was the moment that the terrific quake hit.

"It was a staggering tremor. The car slipped sideways, and then I thought it was going to tip over. *What the heck*, I thought. I hung onto the wheel, opened the driver's door and held it open, with my right foot out to try and stop the car from tipping. People flew out of the disposal facility office, but I saw one woman who couldn't stay upright and had to crawl out on all fours. That's how strong it was."

The Tomioka branch of *Fukushima Minpō* was a one-man local-correspondent operation located in an ordinary house which served both as Kamino's workplace and as accommodation for him, his wife and their three-year-old daughter.

Fortunately, his wife and daughter had moved back to Fukushima city while Kamino spent the last few days busily cleaning and tidying the office in between his usual reporting tasks.

With this sudden and enormous earthquake, he knew from the scale of the motion that there was going to be considerable damage. He dumped the rubbish off at the incinerator and headed back to the office as quickly as he could.

But the road back to the office, which he had just taken in the opposite direction, was now barely recognizable. There were fissures in the tarmac, and in places, half the road had completely subsided. What was left was covered with bumps. All together they demonstrated clearly how the earth had shaken under the immense power of the quake. On top of that, the radio was broadcasting a major tsunami warning.

Above all, he had to get back to the office. Where one lane had subsided he drove tentatively on the other side, nervous that it, too, would collapse under the weight of the car.

Time pressed on relentlessly, but after a number of detours he finally managed to reach the office.

The Tomioka branch of his paper, the *Fukushima Minpō* stood in Block 1 of the Chūō district, the center of town, and about a kilometer and a half northwest of the station. Kamino got his gear together and started on the task of reporting.

The first thing to do in situations like this was to go to the police. The Futaba police station was in the neighboring Chūō Block 2, only three hundred meters to the east. When Kamino arrived in front of the brown three-story building he found an officer shouting, "Get to high ground! You've got to get out of here. It's too dangerous!"

The building, which was old by Japanese standards, having stood there for more than forty years, was still swaying, and with a major tsunami warning now in effect, it was a dangerous place to be.

"Get up on the hill!" shouted an officer he knew. Well, it was a small-town police station and he knew practically everyone there.

Seeing the agitated look on the officer's face, Kamino immediately changed his plans. He knew that the town authorities had created a Disaster Response Headquarters next door to Town Hall, in the Tomioka Art & Media Center up on the hill.

Known as *Manabi no Mori*, 'The Forest of Learning', it was a large community center housing a library, an auditorium, and a local history museum as well as adult education facilities.

As Kamino explained, "The center was equipped with emergency diesel generators, so I knew they'd have electricity even during a power cut. The first floor housed the library and offices, while upstairs were the auditorium and other rooms. It's quite an extensive building."

It was only a kilometer north of the Futaba police station, and for a reporter it was an excellent place to gather information. And that was just what he was expected to do: gather accurate information, edit it and dispatch the result to head office.

When he arrived at the center, Kamino wasn't sure how much time had passed since the earthquake. The upper floor of the two-story building was already bustling in its function as a disaster response headquarters. When he walked in he found the mayor, Katsuya Endō, and his staff there, as well as officers from the police and fire department.

"There's a ship in the middle of the Magata residential community!"

A ship in the Magata community? The Magata community was a developing residential area near Hotokehama beach, a popular local swimming site with a beautiful stretch of sandy coastline, outstanding even among the many beautiful beaches of Fukushima's 'Hamadōri' coast. Travelling north from Iwaki on the Jōban line, the buildings could easily be seen from the train, next to the sea, just before arriving at Tomioka station. And they said there was a boat there.

He couldn't fully grasp what it all meant.

At this point Kamino knew nothing of the tsunami. In getting from the incinerator plant to his office, he had detoured around before dashing to the police station in Futaba and then up here to the disaster response center. What's more, it was still only an hour since the earthquake.

An enormous tsunami must have hit the coast at Tomioka, and if it could carry a whole ship into the Magata community, there was no telling how bad things might be.

Later he was to learn that Tomioka Station, close to Magata, had been swept away, station building and all, leaving nothing but the roof over the platform.

Had the people managed to escape? And what had happened to the buildings?

Astonished though he was, his journalist's habits kicked in and set him to discovering the extent of the damage.

Kamino had in fact prepared for such an eventuality as this and already had a camera spot picked – a bridge over the Tomioka River, with a view south down the coast to the Fukushima Daini nuclear plant.

His responsibilities as a journalist included not only writing, but providing the pictures, too. The head of a local branch of such a regional newspaper had to fulfill all the functions of the office himself, and photography was one of his more important tasks. Now he had not only to write about the actual damage but also photograph the results of the earthquake and the tsunami, all while there was still daylight.

Via numerous detours, he approached the spot near the Route 6, but the scenes he came across before he reached it made him stop the car repeatedly.

There was nothing left of Mayor Endō's home but the storehouse. A former farm, it was a spacious property, but the tsunami had ripped all the buildings out by their foundations. One of the familiar police cars from the Futaba station was sunk in a rice field, with only the upper half of the body visible.

The road was a frightful sight, covered in mud and debris, and littered with signs, lumber, and the wreckage of buildings. The mind-numbing scenes went on and on.

Eventually, just as he was about to reach his photo spot, he was almost stopped by the police. "You can't go any further. It's too dangerous!" shouted the police officer.

He excused himself politely, "*Sumimasen!* I won't do anything stupid!" and pressed on, onto the bridge. The Tomioka River before him was a muddy torrent, and it was flowing *upstream*. The tsunami maintained its amazing momentum.

Kamino clicked away, absorbed in this world of mud. The banks of the river and trees dripped mournfully in this monochrome world. He could barely believe the sights he saw. Even as he took endless shots, it seemed as if the very act of taking photos was but part of a dream.

The scenes before him were like the sepia landscapes of photos of long ago. Everything was buried in the mud, impressing Kamino with the power of the flood.

It was past four o'clock. He could see the Fukushima Daini plant a kilometer and a half away. There was hardly a building left in the foreground, just a few telegraph poles here and there. The rest was a sheet of water. Now it would start to get dark.

Then it suddenly started to snow. Before he knew it, the snow was flying horizontally. The painful cold whipped Kamino's cheek.

"This is what they mean by a natural disaster, I guess," thought Kamino, looking up at the sky. The churning deluge of the Tomioka River and the sudden change in the weather confronted him with the reality that a totally unforeseen catastrophe had struck.

"The snow soon stopped, as suddenly as it had started. Then a strange kind of fog started to flow quickly from the hills toward the sea. It was thin but the color was strong, like nothing I'd ever seen before. The waves rolling up the river met the flow of the returning tsunami, making an unearthly sucking sound. It didn't seem real. It was a creepy sensation."

Video conference

Yoshida roars

Day 1—March 11 Midnight

"What about the iodine? Yes or no!?"

The emergency response center in the earthquake proof building (QPB) at FDI rang with Yoshida's roar.

The executives lined up at the other end of the video-conference, two hundred and fifty kilometers away at the TEPCO headquarters in Tokyo's Uchisaiwai-cho, were startled.

Nearly ten hours after the earthquake, observations of increasing radiation at the plant were making them nervous.

A rising level of radiation could only mean that radiation was leaking from a reactor. If it continued to rise, the building would become unapproachable, which meant it would eventually get out of control.

They had to find a way to get matters in hand before that eventuality.

Yoshida was well-known for his directness. Big and robust, he could hold his drink and go out on the town with his staff: the old-fashioned businessman type. He thought straight, stuck faithfully to his principles and would stand up to his superiors.

In the video-conference, telling-it-like-it-was to the bosses at HQ was where Yoshida shone. His first eruption came in the middle of the night, just after the calendar moved on to March 12.

One of the Tokyo staff who knew what he was usually like, noticing that Yoshida had remained unusually calm and hadn't raised his voice even once since the accident, had commented on

Yoshida's restraint. He spoke too soon. Yoshida was about to display his true specialty for the first time since the accident.

"We've decided to give iodine to those aged under forty, but not to the rest. That's OK with you, isn't it?" Yoshida had asked his superiors in the head office, but their responses were vague and evasive.

"Hey! Make up your minds, will you?"

With Yoshida's demands flying thick and fast, the staff in Tokyo froze. It was Yoshida who had to bear the responsibility for sending his men into the reactor building even though the radiation levels were continually rising.

Iodine tablets are a precaution against uptake of radioactive iodine-131 after a nuclear spill. These tablets are usually taken to provide a measure of protection for workers in contaminated areas.

Usage prescribed by the Nuclear Safety Commission (now the Nuclear Regulation Authority) states that stable isotope iodine tablets are intended only for personnel under forty years of age. It explains that for people over forty years of age there is no recognized risk of thyroid cancer due to exposure to radiation. As a result, at Fukushima Daiichi, instructions had been issued that those aged under forty should take one tablet, while the others would not.

Yoshida had a question. He needed an immediate decision.

"Since radiation levels had been rising since the evening of the eleventh, it was decided that workers entering the plant should take iodine tablets. I asked our radiation control officer, and that was what he said, so I asked him why those over forty didn't need to take them. He told me that that's what the head office had told him, and that it was one of the principles in NSC guidance. But I thought it wasn't fair that, with radiation levels rising, some staff going on site should get the tablets and not others."

Certainly, the grounds for drawing the line at forty were vague.

"Everybody was going in there under the same circumstances and I didn't want any discrimination like that.

"On the other hand, iodine tablets also carry a risk of delayed side-effects in the thyroids. That's what I wanted them to clarify, but the HQ staff responsible wouldn't give us a clear answer. At the time they were in an argument with the NSC over just this point, so they didn't want to issue direct orders. But at our end, I had to send people out into the radioactive site, right away. And time was passing without a decision. That's why I had to get tough with them."

From TEPCO HQ's point of view, they couldn't make their own decision regarding a matter of safety without a definitive reply from the Nuclear Safety Commission. Undoubtedly, they judged that there would be unpleasant consequences if they made a decision without reference to the guidance of the NSC. To Yoshida, this looked like indecision.

In the end, iodine tablets were issued to all those under forty years of age, while the others were given the option to decline them, but this event was to prove only the first instance of a difference in attitude between Yoshida on the site and the headquarters staff in Tokyo.

At this stage, what was most on Yoshida's mind was moving ahead from the need to get some water injected simply to cool the reactors to that of preventing the reactor vessels from exploding. What he needed was a "vent".

"The most important point was how much we could cool the reactors, and what else we could do to make sure the containment vessels were not breached. Anyway, we had to inject some water somehow, but now the diesel pumps weren't working properly, and we didn't have the equipment to inject water. While we were brainstorming, someone suggested we could use fire engines as an alternative."

Fire engines

"The method for injecting water was thought out entirely here on the site," explained Yoshida.

"Using fire engines we could inject the fresh water from local fire cisterns. The idea of using seawater came up, but the difference in level was ten meters and we didn't have any pumps that could handle that. Well, if the fire engines couldn't cope with it, how were we going to get the water up there, we wondered. Then someone realized that, a huge pool, the reversing valve pit in front of Unit 3 (see map page x), remained full of seawater from the tsunami and we decided to use that water first. All this decision-making and brainstorming – 'Let's do it this way', 'No, that won't work. We've got to do it like this,' – this all went on at the plant."

The reversing valve pit was enormous – six point six meters

deep, nine meters wide and sixty-six meters long – and there was one along the front of each unit. For some reason only the pit at Unit 3 was still filled with water from the tsunami. The fire engines were located at the plant's own fire station. A fire engine is basically just a machine that can suck water in and spit it out again, so it should be able to inject water.

"First we can use the water from the fire cisterns. That's what they're there for, isn't it?"

"There's loads of seawater in the reversing valve pit. We could use that. "

On site, ideas were flowing, but to get anywhere near the pit, they'd first have to remove the heaps of wreckage and debris left by the tsunami.

They'd need plenty of manpower for that, because the area around the reactors and vital buildings was heavily fenced as security against terrorism.

As a first step, those fences would have to be taken down to make a route into the area.

The frenzied work went on in the darkness: deciding on a route and getting heavy machinery onto the site to move debris and finally open a route for the fire engines.

Needless to say, the threat of another tsunami and the fear of radiation still hung over the crews. Thanks to their effort, the first water was injected into the reactor around four the next morning. It got there through the pipeline that Hirano and Katō had risked their lives constructing.

At last, more than twelve hours after the tsunami struck, water began to flow into the reactor.

Yoshida recalls, "You might think that pumping some seawater into the system was something that anyone could do, but I assure you it isn't. Some people talk as if it was an easy job, and that really pisses me off. Those people have no idea what we went through, finding a water supply, securing a supply route. They know nothing about it and don't even try to imagine it, but they still think they can lecture about it. It takes longer to actually do it than to just think about it."

However, of the three fire engines at Fukushima Daiichi, two had been wrecked by the tsunami and only one was operable. Finding replacements had become the top priority.

Local Nuclear Emergency Response Headquarters

Confusion

Day 1—March 11 22:00

Out of the lacquer-black darkness, there appeared an endless snow-capped forest. It seemed almost as if the trees had suddenly decided to deliberately loom out of the night.

The hills visible below reached more than a thousand meters. The whiteness of the snow accumulated over the severe Fukushima winter made a stunning contrast with the darkness that seemed to suck them in.

The all-enveloping noise of the helicopter blanketed the ears of seventy-year-old Motohisa Ikeda, deputy-head of the Ministry of Economy, Trade and Industry (METI).

It was past 22:00 on March 11. Ikeda could think of nothing but that they had at last arrived.

"An emergency situation, as defined in Article 15 of the Act on Special Measures Concerning Nuclear Emergency Preparedness has arisen at the Fukushima Daiichi plant." The meeting activating the Nuclear Emergency Response Headquarters (NERH) at METI had started at 16:45. Ikeda had been appointed head and had promptly set off for the site.

Nuclear business operations fall under the jurisdiction of the Ministry of Economy, Trade and Industry, which also supervises and regulates them. One of those operations had met with an unforeseen crisis. Now, as the representative of the government, METI was obliged to provide leadership at the Local Nuclear Emergency Response Headquarters, and to initiate the various procedures that were required. Ikeda was now on his way to take command of the operation.

He'd left the METI building in Kasumigaseki, Tokyo at 17:00. Accompanied by Shin'ichi Kuroki, one of the ministry's deputy director-generals, he'd set off in a ministry car in the direction of Ueno, but had soon become stuck in traffic. Even the capital, Tokyo, had been seriously shaken by the enormous M9 earthquake. Transport was paralyzed, the roads were gridlocked and the minister's car was soon immobilized.

It was at this point that Ikeda, who had to be on-site as soon as possible, requested help from the Japanese Self-Defense Force (JSDF). He set off for Fukushima by helicopter from the Ministry of Defense at Ichigaya, near Shinjuku.

It wasn't until a full five hours later that he was able to alight at the mountain outpost of Ōtakine-yama between Tamura city and the village of Kawauchi, more than forty kilometers west of Fukushima Daiichi.

"It was past ten at night when we reached the JASDF radar station at Ōtakine-yama. It was damn cold! We got into a JASDF vehicle and headed down the snow-covered mountain road for Ōkuma. The road was bumpy and had broken up in places, and we saw houses keeled over, too. The power was obviously out and there wasn't a light to be seen anywhere, or even any sign of life."

On arriving in the disaster area, the severity of the damage made Ikeda stiffen.

The complete blackout left the townships eerily silent. Through the darkness, Ikeda's vehicle headed for the 'Offsite Center' in Ōkuma.

The Offsite Centers (twenty-two nationwide) are designed to serve as bases for operations in response to nuclear accidents. The one at Ōkuma is only five kilometers from the Fukushima Daiichi plant. But when Ikeda arrived there, it was in darkness. (See map page vii.)

"The Offsite Center's diesel generators had broken down. They had no power there, so we went next door to the prefecture's Environmental Radioactivity Monitoring Center building. It was still before midnight. The only means of communication we had was a single satellite phone. I called Tokyo immediately and set to work."

First, Ikeda had to get a grasp of the situation, so he called for a report from the METI nuclear safety inspectors who were still inside the Fukushima Daiichi plant. These nuclear safety inspectors were government officers who, apart from those who were responsible for activating the Offsite Center, were required to stay at the plant to observe and monitor the situation. In what was to become quite a scandal, these government officers would later leave the plant, effectively deserting their posts.

But at the moment, the reports Ikeda received from these inspectors were nothing short of astonishing.

For every single parameter that he wanted to hear—temperatures, pressures, water levels, etc.—the reply they gave him was "No data available."

"How about this? See if you can find that out!" he demanded.

The basic problem was that the control rooms for the reactors had lost all power, so there was no way to even make measurements. It was inevitable that the ministry's safety inspectors had no grasp whatsoever of the situation.

At this point, Ikeda had no idea how bad the situation in the control rooms was. In fact, the only way the operators had of monitoring the parameters was to rig up a small portable generator brought in from outside, wire up a battery to one of the instruments that they wanted to read, and then note the value at that particular moment.

Hold your horses!

Day 2—March 12 01:00

Shortly after 01:00, while Ikeda was still in a flap trying to clarify the situation, a call came in for him, from Tokyo.

"Minister Kaieda is going to hold a press conference at 03:00 about carrying out a vent," he was informed.

In spite of himself, Ikeda parroted back, "A vent?"

This term refers to when some of the steam inside the reactor's primary containment vessel (i.e. not the reactor core itself) is released, or vented, to the atmosphere outside.

Ikeda knew that if the reactor exceeded its safety limits, a vent was necessary to prevent the temperature and pressure from rising and eventually rupturing the vessel, scattering radioactive contamination. But to release the steam pressure from inside even the containment vessel of a nuclear reactor meant contaminating the surrounding area.

This was a matter of public safety. Ikeda began to realize that the scale of the disaster far exceeded his original estimate.

"If the containment vessel were to explode, radioactive material inside would be blasted all over the surrounding area causing terrible contamination. We had to prevent that. If we failed it would be even worse than *the worst ever.*"

What had crossed Ikeda's mind was the Chernobyl disaster.

To avoid that kind of massive release, they would release a limited amount of radioactive steam into the atmosphere, something that had never before been carried out in Japan, nor, on such a large scale, anywhere.

This is what they were up against in order to avoid the ultimate disaster.

Are they really going to do it? Ikeda asked himself.

If TEPCO actually carried out a vent, there would have to be irrefutable reasons to back up the decision.

Ikeda recalled his thoughts of the time.

"It would have been best if we could avoid the vent, but it was essential to stop the containment vessel from blowing up. So I thought we first had to make absolutely sure that a vent was the only way to resolve the situation."

Ikeda explained his view to the staff present at the Local Nuclear Emergency Response Headquarters (henceforth Local HQ) at the Offsite Center in Ōkuma. Masao Uchibori, deputy governor of Fukushima prefecture, and METI deputy director-general Shin'ichi Kuroki were present, along with a party from the Nuclear Safety Commission (NSC). "When I told them what I thought, they reminded me that in this kind of situation, a vent was standard practice. I told them that, even so, as it would affect the safety of the surrounding population, we had to have data to support the procedure before they could carry it out. They gave me the data they had, but it wasn't enough to clarify the problem. So I told them it wouldn't do."

Ikeda summoned the TEPCO team leader and instructed him to collect the necessary data.

"At the moment, the decision to vent has not been made, but

when the pressure inside the containment vessel reaches eight hundred kilopascals (eight atmospheres), the safety valves will automatically open. I reminded myself not to forget that the decision to execute a vent would unequivocally be the responsibility of the company. It was TEPCO's call. Later there was interference from the Prime Minister's Office and all kinds of complaints, but by the rules of organized management, the company and the government were separate entities. It was TEPCO that would make the decision to vent, not the government. The government's responsibility was to make things run smoothly and offer advice when consulted. I realized I mustn't get that the wrong way around.

"I'd been involved with politics for a long time and the incongruity was obvious. This was something the company had to decide for itself."

At this point, Ikeda decided to phone his subordinate, Vice-Minister Kazuo Matsunaga. There was only the one satellite phone and they could rarely get a connection. This severe lack of communications put Ikeda's Local HQ in a very tight spot.

"We could rarely get through on the phone, but we did manage to get through to Vice-Minister Matsunaga and inform him that we were collecting the required data from the plant. I also mentioned that I thought it was inappropriate that the government should be pushing to execute a vent. If the government took too much control over the vent, TEPCO's responsibility would be reduced. That was why the decision to execute a vent would have to be made exclusively by the operator, TEPCO, I told him."

When the TEPCO team leader supplied Ikeda with the data he'd collected, it was almost two-thirty in the morning.

"The report arrived at last. It included such things as figures for the rising pressure in Unit 1 containment vessel. It was going up considerably, and was already over eight hundred kPa. This was twice the pressure at which it was designed to operate. Though it was not my place to make the final decision, now we had been able to obtain real data that showed there was a risk of explosion, I was able to give my permission.

"The designed operating pressure was four hundred and twenty-seven kPa. The pressure had been recorded at a much higher six hundred kPa and continued to rise. Now it had reached eight hundred and forty kPa. If it actually exploded, radioactive material would be spread all over the place. There would be no way to undo that kind of contamination."

It's already past three!!

Day 2—March 12 15:00

At 15:06, Banri Kaieda, minister of METI, accompanied by Akio Komori, the managing director of TEPCO, was attending a press conference in Tokyo.

"We have received notice from TEPCO that since pressure in the primary containment vessel (PCV) is rising, vent valves will be opened to release some pressure," announced Minister Kaieda.

Mr Komori took over, "In order to maintain the safety of the plant, with the esteemed guidance of the relevant controlling agencies, the government, the Nuclear Safety Commission, the Nuclear and Industrial Safety Agency and others, and well aware that this will be of great concern to the inhabitants of the area, we have reached the stage of considering releasing a small amount of pressure from the primary containment vessel."

Release a little pressure? That means letting radioactive material escape from the plant doesn't it? The apprehension among the journalists rose.

Komori explained that they intended to execute a 'wet well vent,' allowing the gas inside the PCV to bubble through water before escaping, but if the situation changed a 'dry well vent,' allowing the gas to escape without filtering through water, might also be considered.

But there was no way the journalists could have grasped the extremely technical and specialized language of his explanation. There was only one thing they wanted to know.

"When will this take place?" someone asked.

Komori replied, "The staff on site have been directed to get things under way around three o'clock."

As it was already past three o'clock, the reporters burst into a hubbub.

"It's already past three!"

"No, three o'clock is just a rough target. They have preparations to make first, and I'll confirm the procedure when I get back there," added Komori.

"Have the residents been informed?"

"It is under way now. I'll check it out when I get back," he answered as the reporters barraged him with questions. Despite the excitement, the journalists could hardly believe the whole thing was real.

Though the foreign term "vent" was new to them, it was quite clear to them that radioactivity was going to be released into the atmosphere.

The message that was taken home by every one of the reporters who took part in the press conference was: *The situation is more serious than we had even imagined.*

Ikeda recalled the press conference with minister Kaieda and TEPCO's Komori.

"While respecting the decisions from the relevant controlling agencies with regard to maintaining safety, TEPCO were going to make a small release of pressure, they said. TEPCO's business attitude just oozed out; they made their point that they were following the agencies' instructions by making just a small release. This is the kind of thing I meant when I talked about having to make TEPCO take responsibility.

"But that's the kind of company TEPCO is. Even though the responsibility is theirs, they don't take their responsibility seriously, you could say. And it seemed that, without doing anything to change that attitude, the government jumped in and took too much control."

At the neighboring Offsite Center, the diesel generators had been repaired and were at last functioning. At 15:17, Ikeda and the staff of the Local HQ were on their way from the Environmental Radioactivity Monitoring Center to the Offsite Center next door.

The situation was galloping on towards the world's first major vent from a nuclear reactor.

The PM's nuclear advisor

Day 1—March 11 19:00

The person who convinced the Prime Minister's Office of the necessity for a vent was the head of the Nuclear Safety Commission, sixty-three year-old Haruki Madaramé. His task was to advise the Prime Minister and the Minister for the Economy on measures to maintain nuclear safety and to handle nuclear emergencies. Though he could not directly control the nuclear operators, his word could literally sway government policy.

At 19:00, four hours after the earthquake, the first steps to respond to the nuclear accident were taken with the establishment of the Nuclear Emergency Response Headquarters at the Prime Minister's Office, with PM Naoto Kan as Director-General and Minister Kaieda as his deputy.

At 19:18 a nuclear emergency was officially declared. Madaramé participated as an advisor.

"After the initial meeting, I popped back to the NSC office inside the Cabinet Office building. I guess I was there for an hour, from about eight to nine that night. During that time I heard how enormous the tsunami had been and began to get an idea of the scale of the damage. But at this point I still assumed they at least had DC power at FDI."

It was a surprise for me to learn that even then, Madaramé, the very person who was expected to advise the Prime Minister, had still not received accurate information. When Chief Cabinet Secretary, Yukio Edano, in accordance with the Nuclear Emergency Act, had declared the nuclear emergency at his press conference, it was still before 20:00.

"I was worried how long their DC power supplies would last. They should have power for at least eight hours, and the tsunami had hit at around three thirty, so eight hours after that, around eleven-thirty that night, that would be when they might get into trouble," recalls Madaramé.

Madaramé envisaged that once the power trucks arrived and were connected, things would be fine.

"With power trucks connected, they would at least be able to keep the batteries recharged, which would give them a break, and once the AC supply was restored, the pumps and other cooling equipment would all be back in action, so I didn't see anything to really worry about."

Then came the shocking news from NISA, the Nuclear Industrial Safety Agency. It was almost 21:00.

"When I heard that the RCIC (Reactor Core Isolation Cooling) system on Unit 2 had stopped I was astonished. I jumped to the conclusion that the batteries that I'd expected to last for eight hours had run down by nine o'clock.

"Well, I expected eight hours and got only five. *Such things happen*, I thought."

In Madaramé's mind, the situation was only as serious as that.

"Nuclear reactors have safety valves, and these valves are always popping open to release steam from the core, so the water inside gradually gets used up. Steam from the core rotates the turbines and the power generated is used to pump water from outside into the core to cool it. That's how the RCIC works."

So, what does it mean when the RCIC is knocked out?

"At the time, this is what I imagined: The RCIC is controlled by DC current, which meant they'd need to use batteries. Those batteries must have run down, and now the RCIC had stopped, I thought. Hypothetically, if the water supply stopped for two hours or so the water level would fall to the tops of the fuel rods, and after another hour, that's three or four hours altogether, the fuel rods would start to disintegrate, and finally the core would melt down. So at this point I imagined we actually had two or three hours to do something about it."

So the core would be on the brink at around midnight, would it? Well, they'll just have to deal with it by then, he'd thought.

"It must have been around nine o'clock. I was informed that Fukushima Prefecture had issued an evacuation order for the two-kilometer zone, and immediately after that I was asked to come to the Prime Minister's Office."

At 20:50, Fukushima Prefecture's Emergency Response HQ had issued an evacuation order for the residents of the area within a two-kilometer radius of the Fukushima Daiichi plant's Unit 1 reactor.

On arriving at the Prime Minister's Office, Madaramé was escorted to a small room on the mezzanine of the national crisis management center. There were sofas and a coffee table in the middle. The room would be cramped with even ten people. METI minister Kaieda was there already, with Eiji Hiraoka, second-in-command at NISA, TEPCO Fellow and vice president, Ichirō Takekuro, as well as Susumu Kawamata, general manager of TEPCO's Nuclear Quality & Safety Management Department.

The room also had two telephones. One of the phones was continuously monopolized by sixty-four-year-old Takekuro talking to TEPCO HQ, while the politicians shared the other. There were other officials coming in and out all the time: Chief Cabinet Secretary Edano, Gōshi Hosono, Tetsurō Fukuyama and Manabu Terata, but the primary instrument for information-gathering was that phone.

"Mr Madaramé," called Kaieda. "TEPCO are asking if *we* can get the self-defense forces (JSDF) to help transport stuff or with evacuating the residents and that kind of thing. You know, the government can't take action at the request of a private company, so I'd be very grateful for your advice," he implored.

The atmosphere was still strained over the prospect of expanding the scale of the civilian evacuation order. But Madaramé didn't know any more about the situation on the ground than Kaieda did himself. They were stranded in a communications vacuum, so to speak.

The lack of information and the pitiful means of communication available to the government's most senior advisor, chair of the Cabinet Office Nuclear Safety Commission, were already becoming painfully apparent.

How far should the evacuation area be expanded? The situation was already as critical as that. Madaramé addressed Takekuro, who was in the room at the time. "Mr Takekuro, it's already that serious, isn't it?"

But Takekuro had no detailed information either. The plant was completely without power, so there was no way Takekuro could have a detailed grasp of the situation, however hard he tried. Takekuro and Madaramé had an exchange of opinions but, unfortunately, Takekuro was unable to supply Madaramé with any concrete information.

One thing that Madaramé had in mind was the figure of three kilometers.

"IAEA policy recommended creating a Precautionary Action Zone (PAZ), so that the local population within a certain pre-defined distance could be evacuated quickly, just in case, even before there was any actual release of radioactivity. If we were worried something might be going wrong, we could warn those people and enable them to escape *before* they were in danger. While the IAEA's recommendation was three to five kilometers, the NSC was still debating the radius. If I remember correctly, this was the moment when I said that, just to be on the safe side, evacuating a three kilometer radius would be appropriate."

At 21:23, orders were issued for the evacuation of residents within three kilometers of Unit 1 at the Fukushima Daiichi plant, and for those within ten kilometers to stay indoors.

This was merely a precautionary measure.

Qualifying his comment carefully, Madaramé responded to Kaieda's request. "Hypothetically speaking, if we lower the pressure in the reactor vessel, it will raise the pressure in the primary containment vessel. We'll need to "feed and bleed" as we release the pressure. That's assuming the residents have already been evacuated, of course."

Feed and bleed? The politicians were at a loss with the unfamiliar foreign words.

"And what, precisely, does that mean," they pressed him. 'Feed and bleed' is a method of removing heat from the nuclear reactor core in the event of an accident by pumping water into the reactor chamber and releasing steam from the valves. It was highly technical terminology, but in the world of nuclear reactors, it was the standard 'first-aid' for cooling in an emergency.

"In short, even if we have to use fire engines or whatever else comes to hand, there is no alternative but to pump water into the reactor."

So they would *feed* water into the reactor and *bleed* off the steam.

But since they'd be releasing steam through the vent valves into the outside world, they'd also be contaminating the surrounding area.

"Here's how I was thinking," Madaramé explained to me. "At that point, even Mr Takekuro didn't know what state the plant was in. But if the RCIC really had stopped then we definitely had an emergency. And if that were the case, then the only thing we needed to think about was how to reduce the pressure in the reactor so they could get some water in, using fire engines or whatever. That was the only thing they could do, I thought, and I'm sure Mr Takekuro agreed."

Clearly, the situation was becoming ever more serious. If things got even worse and the evacuation area were expanded, the politicians would have some hard decisions to make.

"I see," replied Kaieda, looking gravely at Madaramé.

Later Madaramé recalled,

"Though neither Mr Takekuro nor I had sufficient data, we were being asked for decisions and opinions. When I said that if things were as we feared there, then this was the only thing to do, Mr Takekuro agreed. We were of one mind on that."

We *have* to vent.

Day 1—March 11 21:00

This was the first time Madaramé had actually used the word 'vent.'

It was the first time it had happened in Japan, or on such a large scale anywhere in the world, and Madaramé was the first to mention it in public.

"Nowadays, everyone in Japan knows the word 'vent', but when I announced that a vent would be unavoidable, I was the first to use the term. Then, with Mr Takekuro's concurrence, I went on to explain the procedure for executing a vent."

But at that point nobody imagined that there was worse to come.

"At this stage, nine o'clock at night, I was assuming that the fuel rods were intact. So when I explained it, saying 'just to be on the safe side,' I don't think those listening were particularly alarmed. But I remember telling them to hurry because a vent would definitely be required sooner or later. Without a vent there was no way to reduce the pressure. And fire engines wouldn't be able to inject water against a pressure of more than seventy atmospheres. If the pressure inside the reactor reached seventy atmospheres, the only thing to do would be to leak some of it out."

Seated beside Takekuro, who was glued to the phone talking to TEPCO HQ, Madaramé explained things to the politicians: Evacuation was absolutely essential and the vent couldn't wait much longer.

Then things started to take a turn for the worse.

"The flow of information was still fragmental, but the fact that the situation was deteriorating was perfectly clear. The reports that were coming in, though, were often difficult to interpret. For example, they told us they didn't have enough power cables, or though the cables would reach, they couldn't connect them. The plugs were of different types. We didn't know how to make sense of it."

Then Madaramé had a flash of inspiration.

"The report that there weren't enough cables gave me an idea. They should only need a limited number of cables to link to the generator trucks, so they should have more than enough cables on site. I began to wonder if their need for cables meant that the whole power system was down."

Madaramé had been quick to realize that the emergency diesel generators had been flooded, but it hadn't occurred to him that the whole switchboard, deep inside the building, had also been damaged.

"As these reports of a lack of cables came in and I began to think what they needed them for, it occurred to me that perhaps the whole electrical system had been flooded and ruined, so they were having to run cables out to each valve that they wanted to operate. That would be a terrible job. They could never get enough cables for that!"

So the whole electrical power system is out, is it? Madaramé blanched at his own thought.

"Mr Takekuro had worked at the Fukushima Daiichi plant for many years and knew the layout well, but whether or not the switchboard had actually been flooded, even he didn't know. There were all sorts of questions in my mind, but I couldn't find convincing answers to any of them. I remember I had a word with Mr Takekuro, but we couldn't come to a satisfactory conclusion."

Another thing that shocked Madaramé was the rise in pressure inside the containment vessel.

"The most alarming moment was when I heard that the pressure inside the containment vessel had risen to one point five times the design pressure," he said, immediately adding "but it can take that much."

However, the Unit 1 containment vessel was eventually to reach double the design pressure.

"That was the moment that made me think *My God! The fuel rods must have started to melt already!* Among all those people in the mezzanine room in the Prime Minister's Office, only Mr Takekuro and I saw the significance."

What it meant was that the pressure in the Unit 1 containment vessel had reached a level that could occur only if the rods had melted. In that instant, they realized the situation had suddenly turned desperate.

"I remember feeling as if my whole body was on fire, as if a wave of heat ran through me. Whatever happened to me personally after that couldn't be helped, I thought, but it did give me a kind of desperate strength."

Madaramé's mind was thrown into a peculiar state. There was no doubt that the situation was desperate, but the data available to properly assess the situation were still so inadequate. His thirst for knowledge about conditions in the plant was unbearable.

"My mind was full of questions. It's a bit hard to explain, but, for example, with Units 2 and 3 we could pump in loads of water using the RCIC. That water would evaporate into steam, and the steam would raise the pressure abnormally. That I could understand. But Unit 1 was different in that it had an isolation condenser (IC). That means it's fitted with a gravity feed emergency core-cooling system. If this condenser were working, the reactor should cool down, which could only meant that the condenser *wasn't* working. And if it weren't working the reactor should have boiled dry. But if it had boiled dry, then there shouldn't be a rise in pressure. There were so many questions left unanswered."

This was what he'd meant by his earlier "My mind was full of questions."

"There were all sorts of things I was desperate to know, but there was no way to find out. I went through all the physics scenarios that I could think of, but none of them seemed to fit the bill. Nevertheless I was well aware that something very serious was going on."

Though he still didn't have the data to prove it, Madaramé was now convinced that the Unit 1 reactor had boiled dry.

"Radioactivity had probably already escaped. But don't forget there is the containment vessel. I thought it must somehow be holding it in. And I was sure the containment vessel could hold one point five times the design pressure.

"I guess it was a kind of wishful thinking – when people want to believe the best of a situation and convince themselves that it's not as bad as it seems. In fact, the containment vessel will take more than double the design pressure. There have been experiments to prove it, but they were carried out assuming room temperatures. Here the temperature had gone up. How would that change the situation?"

It was past 06:00 and the situation was only getting worse.

"At the very least, the fuel rods must have started to melt inside the pressure vessel. Which meant that a lot of radioactive material must have escaped already, I concluded. I was still pondering the most convincing scenario. At this point, I was stressing that we needed to vent as soon as possible. This was the same thing I'd been saying at nine p.m., but the meaning behind it was now completely different. At a minimum, we had to prevent the containment vessel from rupturing. The urgency was completely different. The politicians kept asking me what needed to be done, but the only answer I had was: 'Hurry up with the vent!'"

Prime Minister Kan had been on the phone to US President Obama since 00:15. In the tiny mezzanine room, discussion continued between politicians, such as Kaieda, Edano, Hosono and Terata, and their technical advisors Madaramé and Takekuro. When he had finished his telephone call with Obama, Kan joined them.

Shortly before 01:00 a message arrived from TEPCO. "The pressure in the containment vessel is extremely high and still rising."

While Madaramé repeated his opinion that there was nothing to do but to vent as soon as possible, Izawa, the shift supervisor at Units 1 and 2, and his staff were already making preparations for that procedure.

I'm in

Shift supervisor

Day 2—March 12 Just after midnight

The tension in the control room located between Units 1 and 2 was steadily rising.

As time went by, all the shift supervisors had assembled in the control room. After Hirano's arrival at 17:00, more staff came in at 19:00 and at 22:00 to offer their support. At 21:00, when the shifts usually changed, all the supervisors and operators from the off-duty shifts were assembled. By this time there were about thirty people in the control room.

But the radiation level was rising mercilessly. There in the darkness, the tedious task of connecting batteries each time they wanted to check an instrument seemed unending.

Since midnight the pressure in the Unit 1 containment vessel had been over six hundred kPa, one and a half times the design pressure.

The expert shift supervisors were of one mind: *We must vent.*

Ever since the evening, while the task of restoring the instruments went on, Izawa and the shift supervisors had been preparing for a vent, running through a checklist of the valves which would need to be opened.

How would they execute the vent? Which valves would be used? Who would operate them?

Without any power, all the valves would have to be opened by hand. Somebody would have to go into the reactor building where radiation levels were steadily rising.

At 23:00 on March 11, about eight hours after the earthquake, intense radiation was recorded outside the double doors at the north entrance to the Unit 1 reactor building, and Site Superintendent Yoshida had declared the reactor building a prohibited area. On the other hand the ERC had told them to confirm the procedure for a vent and the locations of the necessary valves. It was an order to be ready for a vent at any time.

Just after midnight came the order to select the teams to carry out the vent. Izawa and his team in the control room had been working steadily on this long before the order came from the ERC. Their understanding that a vent might become necessary had evolved into a conviction that it was unavoidable.

But when the command came to actually select the teams, it meant a lot to Izawa. "I'll never forget what happened after that order came through," he recalled.

"The procedures that we learn to carry out in case of an emergency always include the possibility of a vent. And having gone through the steps we'd carried out so far, it was obvious to us that a vent was inevitable. But when the time actually came, all kinds of scenes went through my head: my family, the area where I lived. I was already resigned to my own fate but was determined not to gamble with the lives of these operators ranged in front of me. I would send them home alive. That was when the order to select the teams came in. What happened next was unforgettable."

Volunteers

Day 2—March 12 Before 03:00

Izawa finally had to choose his team.

The radiation level in the control room was gradually rising. It was higher on the side near Unit 1, on the right as viewed from the shift supervisor's position. The exhausted operators were sprawled around; some sat in chairs, some huddled on the floor, while others lay as they had collapsed, fast asleep.

"When we checked, we noticed that the radiation was higher away from the floor, so I told them to keep as low as they could. The younger ones were mostly sitting in a circle hugging their knees while a few, who seemed to think that was taking things too far, chose to sit on chairs. The shift supervisors and their deputies mostly stood talking."

Those of shift supervisor rank and their veteran deputies occupied the area in front of the shift supervisor's desk, while the younger operators sat further back.

The light didn't reach the people sitting around walls of the room, so the faces of the people there were invisible.

It was just before 03:00. Izawa opened his mouth.

"Listen up, everyone!"

He took a deep breath and began.

"When we get the go-sign from the ERC we're going to vent. I'd like to select the teams."

A ripple of tension ran through the room.

"I'm sorry, but I can't allow any of the younger men to go. I'd like a show of hands from the rest of you who are prepared to go."

A silence occupied the control room. Everyone stared at Izawa. Not one looked away. His face must have been frozen rigid.

"By this time we all knew that the conditions in the reactor were far from normal. And now, people were going to be sent in there. For us operators, a vent was practically the final card we had to play. And these people would be going in there under my orders. I remember struggling to slowly spit out the words, one at a time," he recalled.

He didn't shout but made his announcement as if telling a story.

For five or ten seconds, nobody spoke. Nobody knew what to say. The silence lengthened until Izawa broke it himself.

"I'll go myself. Will anyone go with me?"

From behind Izawa's left shoulder, Ōtomo spoke out. "I'll go into the building, but you have to stay here, Izawa."

From the other side, Hirano's voice rang out instantly. "He's right. You stay here in command. I'll go."

As the more senior shift supervisors spoke up the junior ones joined in.

"I'll go!"

"Me, too!"

The youngsters broke their silence and raised their hands. As if a dam had broken, the oppressive atmosphere was dispelled.

It was nevertheless gloomy in the control room. There were only a couple of fluorescent light tubes powered by the small generator that they'd brought into the entrance of the service building. Izawa could barely see the expressions on the faces of those who'd raised their hands.

But there was a surprise for Izawa.

"From where I stood, it looked as if it was the junior staff who had raised their hands. Even though we didn't need so many, their hands were up. These were the mid-rank men, barely in their thirties. I was astonished."

Izawa was lost for words. Even though he'd warned them he couldn't allow any of the younger people to go, they nevertheless volunteered.

He was overwhelmed with gratitude. Besides his surprise, he was also filled with a feeling of pride in these people he worked with every day.

"At the time, I just wanted to end it all. Go into the reactor building and get it all over with. Even though we didn't know the exact situation, I'd already sent people inside where things were getting worse and worse. In the end, I'd have to go myself. I felt really bad about it, you know. I just couldn't forgive myself for staying behind while the others went. That's how I felt at the time. When they told me I had to stay in command at the control room, and all the youngsters volunteered like that, my mind just went blank."

Hirano, the one who had told Izawa that he had to stay in command at the control room, had solid reasons for his decision:

"All communication with the ERC came through the same landline and had been handled exclusively by Izawa. He was the one with the most complete grasp of the overall situation at the plant. I thought it best that the person in charge should not be changed. When I arrived at the control room, I'd already decided that I'd make the reactor building my own main responsibility, that's what made me speak to Izawa like that."

Who would make the incursion into the reactor building? he'd wondered.

In these extreme circumstances, each of them was struggling with conflicting emotions.

Izawa was filled to bursting with gratitude, and with contrition, toward the older shift supervisors and the young operators.

Nevertheless, the older men were obviously more familiar with the locations of the valves that needed to be opened and in addition were more suitable for the task simply through being older and less vulnerable to damage from the radiation.

On a whiteboard, Izawa wrote, in order of age, the names of the men who'd volunteered; the shift supervisors, the older men, and those best qualified for the task.

First came the older shift supervisors, Hirano, Ōtomo, Endō and Konno, and then a series of names from the middle ranks, about ten in all, recalled Izawa.

"First, I just wrote out the names and then we discussed who to pair off."

There were two kinds of valve: the MO (Motor Operated) valve, which was normally electrically powered and located on the second floor of the reactor building, and the pneumatic AO (Air Operated) valve, located above the suppression chamber. This latter is a huge donut-shaped cooling device partly filled with water, which is designed to handle excess pressure in the containment vessel. (See diagram page ix.)

The shift supervisors surrounded Izawa, kicked ideas around, and quickly decided their roles.

"I'll do that!"

"That's a job for me."

Altogether there were four shift supervisors and two assistant shift supervisors, a total of six men. The other names disappeared from the whiteboard.

"One said he knew a particular location well, while another foresaw that another part of the route would be physically demanding, so a younger man should go. That was how they settled their roles. There were two locations that had to be visited, so normally two pairs would be sufficient, but if something were to go wrong they would need a rescue team, so a third team was appointed as backup."

Once they'd decided their partners, they had to decide the order in which they'd go in. Ōtomo was first off the mark. "I'll go inside the reactor building," he said. Ōtomo had already been into the reactor building twice: once to actually construct the pipeline and once before that to lay plans for it. This would be his third incursion. His partner would be another volunteer – assistant shift supervisor Tsutomu Ōigawa, aged forty-seven.

The order in which they would go was also decided quickly.

The shift supervisors sorted it out between themselves. Ōtomo and Ōigawa would deal with the MO valve on the second floor, while Endō and Konno went to open the AO valve above the suppression chamber. Hirano, who had been into the reactor building five or six times already – twice into Unit 1, twice into Unit 2 and also to inspect 'the rack' (a set of instruments showing the conditions inside the reactor and the containment vessel) was assigned to the reserve third team.

The tense faces of the shift supervisors in their discussions glowed palely in the light of the generator-powered fluorescent tubes.

All dressed up

Day 2—March 12 04:00

If you are human, it's perfectly normal to feel reluctant or hesitant about entering a building with high radiation levels. But something helped them overcome their fear. None of them has ever explained what it was; whether it was their sense of vocation, a feeling of responsibility, or a fierce determination to protect their families and homes.

Perhaps, even they themselves don't know what it was that drove them. But doubtless each of them conquered his fear in his own way. Izawa, who had been persuaded by his seniors to stay in command in the control room, now had a duty to protect as best he could the men who were actually going to put their lives on the line by going into the reactor building.

"Whatever I did, I had to give them as much protection as possible," he felt keenly. *What can I provide them with?*, he had thought. *That was the most important thing at the moment. If they didn't have the equipment they needed on hand, they'd have to ask the ERC to send it over. And they'd already made numerous requests to the ERC.*

The most important items were full-face masks, SCBAs (self-contained breathing apparatus) and fireproof clothing. These look pretty much the same as what firemen wear when they charge into the flames. They would wear Tyvek suits to prevent contamination through contact with radioactive material, and over that a fireproof suit, with air supplied to the mask from a backpack cylinder.

They'd had all kinds of supplies sent over from the supply depot in the quakeproof building: full-face masks, air-tanks, fireproof clothing and radiation meters. The operators had been into the reactor buildings repeatedly, and each time, their masks and radiation detectors had become contaminated. You might think any full-face mask is a full-face mask, but it was essential to use a *new* one each time they went out!

"Every time anyone went into the reactor building we lost an air cylinder. Each one only lasts about thirty minutes. And we'd been on to the ERC continually, asking them to bring this, and bring that," explained Izawa.

Step by step, preparations went steadily ahead. But the go-sign didn't come. Confirmation that the local people had been completely evacuated had still not come, so they simply had to wait. As the radiation levels rose, so did the strain, as those in the control room awaited the inevitable sortie to execute the vent.

What they didn't know was that the ERC was in uproar as preparations were made for another unforeseen occurrence: a visit to Fukushima Daiichi from the Prime Minister, Naoto Kan.

The PM's Office unhinged

An uninvited guest

Day 2—March 12 04:00

"Prime Minister Kan is coming."

"What?" snapped back State-Minister Motohisa Ikeda, now head of the Local Nuclear Emergency Response Headquarters (Local HQ). He couldn't believe his ears.

It was still before dawn, about four in the morning on March twelfth, at the Local HQ at Ōkuma in Futaba county, only five kilometers from Fukushima Daiichi.

The most important minister in the whole country was about to visit them, right in the middle of an ongoing nuclear accident!

Only hours had passed since Ikeda had arrived and officially set up the Local HQ. What could it mean that the PM was going to drop in?

"After an earthquake and tsunami like that, there were huge numbers of people dead and missing, and the nuclear accident was still in progress. I'd seen some of the footage on TV before I left the ministry in Tokyo, and the scale of that tsunami was simply amazing. The mortality rate for survivors waiting to be rescued from the wreckage would rise severely after seventy-two hours, so the primary focus in those first seventy-two hours should be rescue work. That was standard practice worldwide. I couldn't understand why, in such circumstances, the PM should be visiting the nuclear power station."

It just goes to show how even the leader of the country, the person responsible for the health and prosperity of the whole nation, could be blind to everything but a single small part of the problem.

"The most important thing at that point was rescuing earthquake and tsunami survivors, I thought. The other point was that, even if the PM came to Fukushima, he could attempt to maintain control of the country from there, but land transport and landline communications were wiped out, and so was pretty much everything else. You could hardly get through to anywhere. Even if he came, he wouldn't be able to stay in command, and he'd be better informed about the nuclear accident staying in his office in Tokyo. He needed to maintain a broad overall view, and a balanced one, to keep his priorities straight."

Of course, the nuclear accident was important, but that was all the more reason for the PM to stay in Tokyo where he could maintain the proper perspective, Ikeda thought.

"I told them that if he insisted on coming, then, as his personal safety was of the utmost importance, he should come to the Offsite Center, five kilometers from the plant, in Ōkuma, but in the end I don't think my opinion ever even reached the PM's ears."

At this point, besides Ikeda, sixty-year-old TEPCO vice-president Sakaé Mutō too was at the Local HQ in the Offsite Center. Before 15:30, within an hour of the earthquake, he had left TEPCO HQ in Tokyo and headed for Fukushima in TEPCO's chartered helicopter from the heliport at Shin-Kiba in Kōtō Ward.

Assisting the local government if ever there were a nuclear accident was just one of Mutō's responsibilities.

Regardless, as TEPCO vice-president, he had no doubt that his place was at the Local HQ.

Not that he'd had an easy job getting to Fukushima. Since Japan has severe restrictions on civilian helicopter flights after dusk, he had to reach Fukushima before then. But on leaving TEPCO HQ at about 15:30, he was immediately trapped in post-quake gridlock. He got out of the car and ran.

But Kōtō Ward is land that has been reclaimed from the sea, and Mutō soon got stuck where a road had been damaged by liquefaction during the earthquake. The unusually tall man found himself trapped to above the knees in a quicksand. With the help of passers-by, he was able to escape and, though his clothes were muddied to the waist, he managed to hitchhike two rides, and finally reached the heliport in Shin-Kiba.

The helicopter took off at 17:12 and landed in the grounds

of another TEPCO facility, the Fukushima Daini nuclear power plant at Tomioka in Futaba county at 18:29. (See map page vii.)

After meeting with the head of the plant, Site Superintendent Naohiro Masuda, he left for Fukushima Daiichi, and following repeated detours to avoid the devastation left by the earthquake and tsunami in Tomioka, finally arrived at the plant on the border between the towns of Ōkuma and Futaba around 20:30.

Mutō, who had joined TEPCO immediately after graduation from Tokyo University's engineering department in 1974, stood five years ahead of Yoshida on the promotion ladder, though Yoshida, who had joined the company only after his postgraduate work, was a mere three years younger. They were very close, having spent some time together while posted to Fukushima Daiichi.

"When I went into the ERC, I saw Yoshida busy at his desk, said 'Hi!' and sat down next to him to hear what was up. I learned that the electric power system had been completely wiped out, and more about the situation in the plant. They were barely able to keep in touch with the control room so Yoshida was looking pretty stressed out."

On learning that the Local HQ was not yet in operation, Mutō decided he needed to get out and investigate the local situation. He left FDI shortly before midnight, headed for the town hall in Ōkuma and strode into the Offsite Center in the early hours of the twelfth.

He and Ikeda, head of the Local Nuclear Emergency Response Headquarters got busy getting the Offsite Center in operation, and it wasn't long before the news reached them that the PM was headed for FDI.

Both Ikeda and Mutō were astounded.

"Mr Ikeda stressed that the Prime Minister was a very special figure, not just an ordinary citizen. It was stupid to bring such a vital dignitary to such a place at a time like that, he said. I remember him telling me he'd do all he could to get them to change their plans and stop him from actually visiting the plant. For my own part, I was concerned that if the PM actually deigned to pay us a visit, as a TEPCO vice-president I'd have to express my apologies and explain the situation to him."

At this point the Prime Minister's Office in Tokyo was still in turmoil as they made preparations for the trip.

Haruki Madaramé, head of the Nuclear Safety Commission, was informed by one of the prime minister's staff, out of the blue, that it had been decided that the PM would visit FDI, and would Madaramé please accompany him? That was at 05:00 in the morning.

At the sudden summons, Madaramé was at a loss.

"I wasn't told until about an hour before departure and without any warning. It was quite a shock. What use was it for *me* to go? I couldn't understand it. I couldn't drive a fire engine or anything, and the people on the ground understood the situation better than anyone. More importantly, why was the PM himself going? That was incomprehensible."

Madaramé tried to get more information from the PMO staff.

"Why do you need *me* to go?" he asked.

"On your way to the site, the PM would like you to explain in more detail. You can accompany him and fill him in before you arrive," he was told.

Ah, so that's it, is it? thought Madaramé. The PM wanted the inside story from him personally. In that case, he had to go. He'd had hardly a word directly with Kan about the accident so far.

Like a game of Chinese Whispers, it was always someone else that had passed on Madaramé's opinions to the Prime Minister. If the PM now wanted to hear directly from him in his role as advisor, there was nothing for it but to tag along, he realized.

First, he accompanied the PM to the third floor of the building, where the media were waiting. At the press conference there, Kan announced his intention to visit the FDI site, taking care to point out that he would have a nuclear power expert to accompany him. That was Madaramé. It was all happening before his very eyes. He had hardly had any contact with the PM since the accident, and was left with a peculiar feeling as Kan spoke to the journalists.

Madaramé recalled that there had been a scene earlier, on the way to the press conference on the third floor, when Edano, the Chief Cabinet Secretary, had yelled to Kan in the corridor from the national crisis management center, "Prime Minister, you must designate an acting prime minister!"

Besides his role as head of the national crisis management center, PM Kan was also head of numerous other organizations.

While the PM was absent from his post, Edano would be left in charge and had every right to request that he be given full executive powers.

"I hear you," Kan snapped back.

Numerous parts of the Prime Minister's Office are closed to journalists, including the national crisis management center and the elevator to the roof, but as Kan stepped into the elevator after the press conference, his grim expression remained unchanged.

Shortages

Day 2—March 12 05:00

On hearing that the PM was on his way, Yoshida was perplexed. The leader of the entire nation was coming to visit their contaminated battlefield. If he actually arrived, they'd have to make sure he was sufficiently prepared, both mentally and materially. They'd need to take strict measures to prevent any contamination.

"I think it was about five in the morning when we first heard about the prime minister coming. We weren't told *when* he would come until just before he arrived. We had to decide where his helicopter could land and, once it had landed, how to get him from there to the ERC in the quakeproof building, and we only got that worked out shortly before his flight took off," Yoshida recalled.

"The helicopter would land on the sports ground to the west of the quakeproof building. Once they'd put it down on the landward side, we would escort the PM into the ERC. This is where I got into a bit of a scrap with TEPCO HQ."

The problem centered on the full-face masks that the visitors were to use. For the visit of the prime minister and his party to the contaminated area, Yoshida, as Site Superintendent, wanted to be sure everyone wore a proper mask and protective gear. However, they didn't have enough spare equipment at the plant.

"At our end, we were fighting desperately to restore the plant. Every time someone went into the reactor building they used a mask. That then got contaminated, and a new one was required. Spares? We hardly had enough for ourselves! Every item was accounted for."

That was how Yoshida put it. And now they had to provide for people who would do nothing to help to restore the plant. They couldn't afford to share their equipment.

"That was when I asked HQ in Tokyo over the video link to have them bring their own equipment. But they insisted that we had to find the stuff on site. We didn't have enough gear at the plant; I mean, we were already recycling parts to make new sets of gear. I told them we didn't have anything to spare. It wasn't as if the PM was coming all by himself, after all. HQ told me again we had to find the stuff on site, and I lost it and shouted that they were out of their damned minds."

If they really didn't have the stuff in Tokyo, Yoshida was the kind of person who was prepared to tell them "Improvise," or "Look again. You'll find something somewhere." In the ERC at FDI they were frantic, trying to cope with the situation. They couldn't spare equipment that they needed on site just to welcome the Prime Minister and his entourage.

"The reactors were the most important thing as far as we were concerned. At that point, we were right in the middle of wracking our brains trying to work out how to bring the vent forward. We were up to the eyes in work, constantly checking the situation in the reactor building, finding out what bottlenecks were holding things up and what we could do to clear them. The security team could meet Mr Kan and his party and show them around, I told them. Preparations for the vent were the responsibility of a completely separate work group. They were different teams, so I asked them to make sure that things *stayed* separate and that everything went smoothly."

It's clear that Yoshida, who was already heavily burdened with the vent and numerous other tasks, honestly had no resources left to welcome the Prime Minister and his entourage.

"I'd given instructions to the head of the recovery team to report regularly and make sure that nothing got in the way of operations. But as far as preventing the visitors from coming, there was nothing more I could do."

And if the visit meant that the inside of their frontline command post, the ERC itself, were contaminated, the battle would be lost, Yoshida thought.

"If the party got contaminated outside they would become a source of contamination themselves, so we couldn't have them enter the quakeproof building, could we? But they just said "So what?" and played even more stubborn. I've a suspicion that Mr Kan didn't even realize that he himself could actually get contaminated. I don't think he had a clue about things like that. He simply wanted to get inside the ERC and hear all about it as soon as possible, so he came. He didn't deliberately make a nuisance of himself. It was just plain ignorance on his part. From that point of view, I wish the experts had told him more beforehand."

Super Puma

Day 2—March 12 06:00

On the roof of the Prime Minister's Office, built at a cost of seventy billion yen, with five stories above ground as well as a basement, there stood a helipad. In case of emergency, the pond in front of the building could be drained to form another helipad, but normally only the one on the roof was used.

The press conference on the third floor was over in a matter of minutes and the prime minister's party bustled its way to the roof. The helicopter was a Super Puma, reserved for VIPs. The upper parts were silver and the lower parts grey, a smart look, with the Japanese characters for Ground Self Defense Forces in black.

When the Super Puma carrying Prime Minister Naoto Kan roared into the sky on its way to FDI it was 06:14 on the morning of March 12, 2011.

The Super Puma had been in the public eye before when it was used to carry heads of state of the industrialized nations to the Tokyo Summit. Behind the pilots there were two rows of seats separated by an aisle. It could carry about ten people at a time.

The atmosphere inside the helicopter was painful. The PM's irritation knew no bounds, and since the previous evening he had been blasting the staff of the PMO and his ministers alike with withering comments.

The PM sat on the left hand side facing forward with his Special Advisor, Manabu Terata, opposite, while to the PM's right across the aisle, sat Madaramé.

"It was March, so it was pretty cold. I was still wearing my long-sleeved underwear under my shirt every day. And I had my Nuclear Safety Commission jacket on over that. In the helicopter,

Kan sat down on the left facing the front and I took the seat on the right separated from his by the aisle. So there I was, side-by-side with Kan, and with only the aisle between us. I think it was his Special Advisor, Terata, who sat opposite him. We were sat in pairs facing each other. Some other people boarded after us so there were about ten in all."

Kan's expression was grim. He'd been demonstrating his famous ill-temper since the previous evening, castigating his underlings left, right and center, and there was no change in his look when he boarded the helicopter.

Intending to impress the prime minister with the gravity of the situation, Madaramé started to explain. After all, he had been brought along specifically for the purpose of filling him in on the details.

"There was no need for me to explain to him anything so elementary as that there was no risk of a nuclear explosion, but he needed to know about the problem of decay heat, so that's where I started. I was going to tell him how, in a situation like this, the decay heat was enormous, and that if water was not injected into the reactor, a catastrophic meltdown like the "China Syndrome" scenario was a real possibility. Well, that's how you'd start with a normal person. But as soon as I started to explain he interrupted, and with an attitude of 'I know that already,' told me flatly to simply answer his questions."

'Just answer my questions!' The finality of Kan's words struck Madaramé dumb. Despite this being a perfect opportunity to consult an expert directly, it was about to degenerate into a mere string of responses to Kan's questions.

"What's the difference between the reactors at Units 1, 2 and 3?" asked Kan. A basic question. Madaramé explained, "The power output is different. Unit 1 is rated at four hundred and sixty Megawatts while Units 2 and 3 can produce seven hundred and eighty MW. They're totally different. Unit 1 is a BWR/3 type while Units 2 and 3 are BWR/4s. Unit 1 has an emergency condenser called an IC to cool it down, but Units 2 and 3 have RCICs which cool the reactors by injecting water. The IC is considered more reliable since its circulation depends on convection, so it's odd that things should turn out like this," he added.

"Why does Unit 1 have an IC when Unit 2 has an RCIC?" asked Kan.

"Because the power output is so much higher in the later model, the natural convection in the IC is not sufficient to cool the larger reactor, so the system was changed to one that has a turbine to pump in water, I believe," replied Madaramé, as he began to realize that Kan did have some grasp of the problem.

"What happens if the fuel rods melt?" Kan continued.

"If the fuel rods melt, the cladding made of a zirconium alloy known as Zircaloy, being a metal, reacts with water at high temperatures and releases hydrogen."

"What's going on now?"

"I imagine the hydrogen will have reached the containment vessel by now."

"If hydrogen gets out, it'll explode, won't it?"

"No, it won't. Even if hydrogen gets out into the primary containment vessel, the PCV is filled with nitrogen, so there's no oxygen there and it can't explode. When we conduct the vent, the hydrogen will reach the top of the chimney and come in contact with air for the first time, where it will just burn up," answered Madaramé. It was an extremely technical discussion. The question of whether or not the hydrogen would explode was not a question that you'd expect to spring to mind in a layman. Kan had more than a little prior knowledge of the topic.

Madaramé remembers this question-and-answer session vividly.

"We went through all the steps in order. And I answered everything I was asked."

One point in this interchange was later taken up and became the subject of widely spread rumor, namely the assertion that it wouldn't explode.

Kan and Madaramé's dialogue about hydrogen merely affirmed that the containment vessel itself wouldn't explode. If the containment vessel did explode, it would lead to a situation that was too horrifying to imagine.

Though what they discussed was of a completely different level, when the outer shell of the reactor building was blown off, Madaramé was subjected to severe criticism.

At last they neared their destination.

"Aren't there any nuclear power experts at Titech?" asked the PM.

This was an unexpected question. For a moment, Madaramé was stumped. Why on earth should the prime minister ask whether there were any nuclear power experts at the Tokyo Institute of Technology?

But then he recalled that Prime Minister Kan was himself a graduate of Titech.

"That's when it came back to me: *Ah, yes, he's from Titech himself!* So I suggested the names of two more Titech graduates. But one of those had gone on to work for TEPCO, so I told him several more."

The fact that Kan called on his contemporaries and fellow alumni from Titech to advise the Cabinet in this time of emergency is now well known. Whether it was from an extreme loyalty to his old school, or that he could not trust people from other colleges, it shows that Kan had an unusual way of thinking.

"What's that?" Kan quizzed Madaramé afresh.

Their helicopter was flying over the sea. Looking out of the window behind Kan's back, Madaramé spotted the chimneys of a power station. It was the Hirono thermal power station in Futaba county, roughly twenty kilometers south of FDI.

"I could see the station over Kan's shoulder, so I told him it was the Hirono thermal power station. I'd been looking out over the PM's shoulder and thinking that we must already be over Iwaki, so when I saw the chimneys I knew immediately where we were. I'd often been up this way so I knew the area. Once we saw the plant at Hirono, it wasn't far to Fukushima Daiichi. And sure enough, FDI soon came into view." (See map page vii.)

I asked him how they each felt on seeing this view. At this point it wasn't the appalling sight that it was soon to become when the upper part of the reactor building was blown off by a hydrogen explosion. The white buildings were neatly arranged amongst the greenery. The deep blue of the sea, and the plant itself amid the deep green of the surrounding woods made an impressive sight.

However, as the helicopter's descent toward the landing ground brought them closer, they became aware of the scars of the tsunami. The reactors, the oil tanks and other buildings lined up along the shoreline stood surrounded by wreckage. Wordlessly, the spectacle portrayed the immense power of the tsunami.

But they had no time for sentiment. There was a battle going on down there, with lives being risked to restore the plant.

After the helicopter had landed and Madaramé was preparing to alight, something happened which really annoyed him. A voice announced, "Please remain in your seats until the Prime Minister has disembarked."

The rest of the party were not allowed to disembark immediately. Prime Minister Kan's visit to the stricken site was no more than a photo op! *What nerve!* thought Madaramé. *A photo break? At this critical moment in the fight to save the plant?*

Kan vents

Day 2—March 12 07:00

The party appointed to welcome the PM (consisting of Local HQ chief Motohisa Ikeda, Vice-Governor of Fukushima Prefecture Masao Uchibori, Vice-president of TEPCO Sakae Mutō and Deputy Director-General of METI Shin'ichi Kuroki), awaited the arrival of the helicopter on the sports ground at FDI. Ikeda and his companions, who had driven the five kilometers from the Offsite Center in Ōkuma, watched the approaching helicopter in silence. They were standing in a contaminated area. (Site ②, page viii.)

Mutō had originally intended to go to the ERC and hear what had happened overnight directly from Yoshida before going to greet the Prime Minister.

"First, I went to the QPB, but because the area was already contaminated, they were scanning everybody who came into the building, one by one. There was a huge queue. I guess I could have pulled rank and jumped the queue, but if I waited in line I'd be late, so I did a U-turn. There wasn't much time, so I drove straight to the sports ground to wait for Mr Kan's helicopter."

Mutō managed to exchange a few words with fifty-two-year-old Masaru Sekiya, one of the staff who was scanning people for radioactivity at the entrance to the QPB. Sekiya was manager of the Radiation Safety group at TEPCO's Kashiwazaki-Kariwa Nuclear Power Plant in Niigata.

Sekiya, an expert on radiation control, had been employed at FDI until two years earlier. When the huge earthquake occurred, he had formed an expeditionary support team at Kashiwazaki-Kariwa, had reached FDI in the middle of the night, and had immediately initiated a radiation control program at the quake-proof building, where radiation levels had already started to rise. His team was currently composed of staff from both Kashiwazaki-Kariwa and Fukushima Daichi power plants.

"How are we supposed to get the PM here?" Mutō asked Sekiya.

"Stop the bus right here by the entrance and get them inside as quick as you can," Sekiya answered. That was the only way to keep their exposure to radiation as low as possible.

Sekiya recalled, "Actually, we'd already been asked to measure the background radiation at the ground where the helicopter would land. They wanted us to check beforehand whether the sports ground was contaminated, and if so how badly. The PM was going to walk in his own shoes, so they wanted us to check if there was any radioactivity there before he arrived, but he and his party arrived before I heard the results. They were so busy handling the accident itself that they weren't able to prepare for the visit before the entourage arrived. That the Super Puma could reach there from Tokyo in under an hour was an impressive demonstration of its speed."

At this point, Mutō tried to call Yoshida from the landing ground.

"I'd not been able to ask about the situation since the night before or to even see Yoshida before arriving at the landing ground. In fact, I was the first to arrive. I thought I'd phone Yoshida from my mobile but I couldn't get through. Fortunately there was a security vehicle there and I was able to persuade the crew to let me use its radio. I asked them where I could get through to and they told me it was linked to the ERC, so I got them to call Yoshida for me. I told him I was at the landing ground and was about to bring the PM to the ERC, so could he prepare a meeting room? Yoshida said he'd see to it."

So, Mutō had no choice but to meet the PM without learning any more about the situation than what he'd heard the night before. Eventually, Ikeda and Kuroki joined him at the sports ground. And soon the helicopter carrying Kan arrived too.

Looking as grim as ever, Kan disembarked and came toward them. Ikeda said, "He looked at me and I think he said 'Hey, there!'

or something like that." But when Mutō went to greet him the atmosphere changed abruptly.

"Mutō from TEPCO, sir. It's very kind of you to come," he introduced himself deferentially, but Kan's response was to bark back, "Why haven't you vented yet?"

What? thought Muto.

Mutō wasn't the only one to be astonished. Everyone there was astounded to hear Kan bellow at Mutō without so much as a greeting.

Kan was furious. Perhaps it was simply that a suitable victim had at last appeared before him.

So, his first words to the tall vice-president of TEPCO, on the radioactively contaminated sports ground at FDI, were "Why haven't you vented yet?"

Right next to Ikeda stood Satsuki Eda, who, having been involved in the formation of the Social Democratic Party of Japan's policy study group, *Sirius,* (1992) had known Kan for almost twenty years and had experienced quite a few of his explosive bouts. But he hadn't expected that as soon as he had debarked from the helicopter he would vent his anger on Mutō like that.

"After that, we all got straight on the bus. The PM sat in the second row on the right, behind the driver, and next to TEPCO's Mutō. I sat on the left, across the aisle, and I had Madaramé sit behind the PM. The seating was my responsibility. But the PM's fury was worse than usual."

On the left and to the rear, Ikeda was unable to catch what the PM actually said.

"He was furiously yelling something at Mutō, spitting out words like a machine gun, but his tone was so fierce I couldn't make out what he said," he remembered, recalling the scene on the bus.

Even in the seat behind the PM, Madaramé said, he was unable to make out what he said. "I couldn't figure out what he was saying either. He was raging on at Mutō about something but he was gabbling so wildly, I couldn't follow what it was all about"

Kan's mood was clearly different from when he was in the helicopter. He must have boiled over on reaching the site.

Mutō reflects "The very first thing he said was 'Why haven't you vented yet?' and then he wanted to know why we hadn't vented earlier, when we would be executing the vent, why we couldn't do it now, and the like, repeating the same questions over and over. I can't forget how he kept claiming he wanted to know what the problem was, but had no intention of listening, and just went on bellyaching that we weren't doing our job."

In about three minutes, the bus arrived at the QPB and drew up alongside the main entrance. Mutō had arranged beforehand with Sekiya where to stop the bus – as close as possible, only two or three meters from the doors.

The building had two sets of automatic doors. First, the outer doors were opened, people entered the sixteen square meter 'air-lock', the outer doors were closed, and then the inner ones opened, ensuring that in case the air outside was contaminated as little as possible would get into the building.

However, the previous day's earthquake had distorted the doors, and, because of the power blackout, they had to be operated manually. Sekiya was responsible for opening and closing the doors, and with two more men for each door and a few "Heave-hos!" to help him, they hauled them open and shut.

There, the Prime Minister arrived. Leading the way was Mutō, who had been so badly abused on the bus. He stood a head taller than the rest. With him at the head, and with Kan, Ikeda, Madaramé and Kuroki close behind, the party of slightly more than a dozen dashed past the manually opened outer doors into the space inside.

"OK! Open up!" Sekiya shouted, once he had made sure they had everyone safely inside. The inner doors were heaved open and he waved the group inside.

Inside the entrance of the building there was a corridor about two meters wide which ran straight through to the back of the building. The stairs were to the left, but first Sekiya had the party move down the corridor.

There they found a team of radiation inspectors waiting. Each of the visitors needed to be checked for contamination before they could be allowed upstairs.

The stern-faced Kan ignored Sekiya's "Good morning, sir."

"Please remove your shoes and carry them in your hand," Sekiya asked the group. "Down the corridor are the radiation inspectors. First, please let them examine you for contamination," he continued. They started to move down the corridor for the inspection, but an angry voice rang out.

"What do you think I came here for? There's no time for this nonsense!"

The voice reverberated throughout the floor. Its owner; none other than Prime Minister Kan himself. It seems he found the thought of being subjected to an inspection objectionable.

I've no time for an inspection! What do you think I came here for? The crowds of employees returning to the building from work on site were astonished.

Ikeda, who was near Kan at the time recalled "*This is awful,* I thought. There were operators all down the side of the corridor, some of them naked to the waist. Right in front of these operators, who had just returned from recovery work inside the reactor building and were waiting to be inspected for contamination, there he was, bellowing 'What do you think I came here for?' The Prime Minister himself comes, and instead of lauding the employees for their efforts, he's shouting things like that? It was just too awful."

The people around him flinched at his ferocity. There was no way they could inspect him for contamination now.

"Please leave your shoes here and change into these."

Sekiya nimbly changed the subject and requested them to change into a pair of the 'blue shoes' that were worn inside the ERC. They obeyed silently and slipped them on. Then Mutō led the party up the stairs to the left of the entrance, to the second floor.

Kan and Yoshida

Day 2—March 12 07:20

The party went up the stairs, turned right along the corridor and filed into the last room on the right. There were conference tables in the middle of the room, but the room was barely big enough to hold them all.

Kan sat at the end on the right. Ikeda, Madaramé, and Kuroki took the seats next to him. The seat opposite Kan was taken by Mutō. Yoshida had not yet arrived.

"Why don't you get on with the vent?"

There was only another minute to wait until Yoshida arrived but Kan resumed his attack on Mutō.

When Mutō tried to reply, he was harshly brushed off.

"I didn't come here to hear that kind of nonsense."

That was when Yoshida walked in. He was a little late, because making arrangements with the people down in the control room had taken longer than expected. From the ERC, moments before, he had told them, "I'm going to meet with the prime minister now, but if anything comes up, don't hesitate to interrupt."

"Site Superintendent Yoshida, sir," he introduced himself. Prime Minister Kan versus Masao Yoshida. It was the first time they'd met.

Kan had graduated from the Applied Physics department of Titech (Tokyo Institute of Technology) in 1970. Yoshida, who had graduated from Titech in 1977, had gone on to postgraduate studies, so Kan was, by Japanese customs of seniority, his '*sempai*' by seven years.

Kan, who had been berating Mutō, now turned to Yoshida, who had sat down on Mutō's left. The first words out of his mouth were, "What the hell is going on?"

To those around them, it seemed as if the barrage directed at Mutō had simply shifted to Yoshida.

Yoshida responded, "Even though there is a total power blackout, we are trying everything we can to proceed with the vent, but conditions in the reactor building are making things difficult."

He tried to explain the details of the situation but Kan interrupted.

"How did it get like this?" His fury had not subsided in the least.

"Well, it's like this," replied Yoshida, spreading out a plan of the plant he was holding. "Please take a look," he said, showing it to Kan. "This area was flooded by the tsunami. The water got inside the buildings and consequently we lost all power. The pumps and motors are all in the basement, so they were all flooded and disabled, and remain inoperable."

Kan had begun to listen to Yoshida's careful explanation.

"We've managed to keep a few of them ticking over, but most of the ECCSs (Emergency Core Cooling Systems) which cool the reactor cores are out of order," he continued. He simply had to get the PM to understand the severity of the situation.

"Hadn't you planned for that?" asked Kan. From the atmosphere in the room, Yoshida realized at this point that because of Kan's fury, no one else in the room had the nerve to as much as slip a word in edgewise.

Again he explained how this tsunami, of unforeseen size, had engulfed essential buildings even on the ten-meter level. Yoshida was the kind of person who, in his normal day-to-day work, would speak his mind even to the higher ranks. On this occasion too, he gave Kan a candid explanation. Ikeda, head of the Local HQ described how he remembered the dialogue.

"I had heard that the many of the staff at TEPCO were a Machiavellian lot but Yoshida gave a completely different impression."

Madaramé who had also been present recalled his impression.

"At first, Mutō had done his best to answer Kan's questions but had been angrily told 'I didn't come here to hear that kind of nonsense!' After that, Yoshida came into the room and took over. The focus moved to Yoshida and Kan, and Kan actually listened to what Yoshida had to say."

Eventually the question with which Kan had belabored Mutō was turned on Yoshida.

"What's going on with the vent?"

Yoshida replied, "We are working on it. However, as we have no power, the electrically operated valves need to be opened manually, so conditions in the reactor building continue to make things difficult. Work is going on inside the building to get those valves open at this very moment."

Didn't Kan already know that there was radiation inside the reactor building and that it was necessary to work by hand, in the dark? Well, now Yoshida had explained it to him in detail.

"More than anything, you must get that vent done as soon as you can," demanded Kan. Of course, Yoshida and his staff had already been working on the problem for some time. However, at this point they were still waiting for confirmation that the local population had been evacuated.

"We are doing everything we can, of course. We also have a suicide squad ready."

At these words, Kan seemed to calm down a little. The tense atmosphere that had surrounded him had somewhat relented.

At this point, METI Deputy Director-General Kuroki, who

had come with Ikeda from the Local HQ, addressed the prime minister.

"Prime Minister, would you sign these, please?" he asked, quickly offering him a couple of documents.

These were the declaration of a separate nuclear emergency at the Fukushima Daini nuclear power plant and the order for the evacuation of civilians from a three-kilometer radius around *that* plant, for which he needed the PM's approval. This provided a moment's breathing space.

"These will do," commented Kan, as he looked over and signed the documents.

Ikeda later explained, "Things were getting a bit odd at the Daini plant too and we thought an evacuation might become necessary, so Tokyo asked me to get those signed. If the PM had stayed in Tokyo, it could have been done immediately, but since he had come to Fukushima, it was left up to me. As head of the Local HQ, it wasn't my responsibility, but that of Kuroki, the METI Deputy Director-General. Strictly speaking, *he* was supposed to do it. That's why he'd brought the documents and come to meet the PM's helicopter as soon as it landed. But the PM was in such a rage that Kuroki couldn't find a suitable moment to address him. Getting his signature could have been done in the bus, or anywhere. So from that point of view, the time lost there caused a delay in the issue of the evacuation order."

Ikeda commented that at Yoshida's use of the term 'suicide squad' in relation to the vent, Kan had calmed somewhat, and that had provided the opportunity to get his approval.

"That Yoshida was an imposing figure, fearless, and when he put it straight to the PM, he actually got him to listen. When Yoshida used the phrase 'suicide squad', it stunned him, well, enough to calm Kan down a little."

The PM and his entourage left the Emergency Response Center at 07:42. His conversation with Yoshida had lasted about twenty minutes.

Carrying out the vent involved going into the darkness of the radioactive reactor building and opening the valves by hand. Hearing the word 'suicide squad' seemed to have made Kan realize that the sortie into the radiation of the reactor building marked the actual start of the vent, and he must have been relieved.

Leaving the ERC and descending the stairs to the first floor, Kan put his hand on Ikeda's back and encouraged him with the word '*Gambatte!*' The PM seemed a bit calmer now. But Ikeda himself had something to say to the much younger Manabu Terata, Special Advisor to the Prime Minister. "Terata, my boy, try and calm him down, will you?"

Terata, only thirty-four years old, and already a representative in the Lower House, belonged to Kan's own wing of the Social Democratic party and had been personally appointed Special Advisor by Kan. Ikeda, a member of the cabinet himself, was entrusting the task of calming the enraged Prime Minister to the PM's own protégé.

In the cold of the early morning they had trouble re-starting the engine of the helicopter. Ikeda, Uchibori and Mutō remained standing amid the contamination of the sports ground waiting for it to take off.

When the helicopter carrying the prime minister and his entourage lifted off to inspect the earthquake and tsunami damage in neighboring Miyagi Prefecture, it was four minutes past eight in the morning.

Kan's defence

Kan was later severely criticized for the chaos caused by his visit to the plant. In October 2012, a year and seven months after the accident, he recalled the event to the author.

"At the time, TEPCO sent Mr Takekuro to liaise with the Prime Minister's Office. Takekuro had risen to become one of their vice-presidents, responsible for nuclear power and plant siting, so he was an expert on nuclear power, a real veteran. That's why they sent him. Of course I had lots of questions for him about the situation. But he couldn't explain what was going on. At one point he told me that if things went on as they were going, there was a danger that the pressure in the containment vessel would keep rising until it exploded, so they wanted to conduct a vent, and he wanted my consent to that. So I said, Okay. But even though they said themselves they were going to vent, nothing happened. When I asked him why, he couldn't answer. He hadn't received the necessary data. There *was* no data. TEPCO HQ must have had the answers, so why didn't they pass them on to Mr Takekuro? If he couldn't explain how things stood, what do you expect me to do but ask them 'Hey, what's going on?' That was why, when I met Mutō at the plant, I asked him straight out, 'What's going on?' It was a perfectly natural thing to ask, from my point of view!"

Kan confirmed that the first person to satisfactorily explain the situation to him was Site Superintendent Yoshida.

"Yes, that's right. That was the first time that we'd met. He seemed to me to be a man with guts, and until we met, I'd no idea we were from the same college. He was very clear and easy to understand.

"He'd say 'This is what we want to do, and this is how we are doing it.' So in a very short time he was able to tell me, nice and clearly, what they were doing and why. That was fine with me. If he'd gone into more detail, I wouldn't have understood it anyway. Nobody had ever tried to explain things to me like that before. He managed to convince me that he knew what was going on, and that was fine with me, so I left him to it."

As far as the prime minister was concerned, he hadn't been able to find anyone who could describe the circumstances convincingly until he reached the plant.

"Whether it was to do with the vent or the situation at the nuclear plant, when TEPCO wanted something done, there was always someone to advise me. At that time, for example, it was Madaramé, head of the Nuclear Safety Commission. So whenever there was a decision to be made, I'd get to hear TEPCO's point of view.

"As well as that, there was NISA (the Nuclear and Industrial Safety Agency), of course, as they make up the secretariat of the Nuclear Emergency Response Headquarters, and if their experts or someone who knows had something to tell me, I'd listen to their opinions. I'm always listening to their advice. As for all this talk about me thinking that I know it all, and telling them to do this and do that, I can assure you, there is no truth in that whatsoever. If, at that time, the reason they couldn't do the vent was that they couldn't confirm that the civilians had been evacuated, then they should have said so, shouldn't they? If the radiation was too high so the work was more difficult than they'd expected, or the manuals said so-and-so, or whatever, if they'd at least had some explanation . . . At any rate, there was nothing like that. How was

I supposed to know any more than that if they didn't tell me? That was why I went to the plant."

So, from Prime Minister Kan's point of view, the visit to the FDI was the natural thing to do.

But, either Mr Takekuro or Deputy Chief Cabinet Secretary Tetsuro Fukuyama *had* informed him of the difficulties of a manual vent and the delays due to the rising levels of radiation.

It would seem that the root of Kan's decision to visit FDI lay in a fundamental distrust of TEPCO that he had held from the start.

"It's all because TEPCO didn't explain themselves properly. The vent, for example; at one o'clock they said they were going to do it, but at three o'clock they'd made no progress. Mutō too; he may have known what was going on, but he just mumbled on without actually explaining anything. If you want to talk about mistrust, then there's the reason. I mean to say, at a time like that, the two top dogs (Tsunehisa Katsumata, TEPCO chairman, and Masataka Shimizu, President and CEO) were off on a trip. We needed them to make some kind of decision. If Mutō were such an expert, if he thought he had the answer, he should have stepped up and told me his professional opinion."

That is how Kan recalled his visit during the chaos.

Saving the day

Stop and go

Day 1—March 11 18:00

The 6th Artillery Regiment of the 6th Division of the Japan Ground Self-Defense Force is stationed in the city of Kōriyama, sixty kilometers west of the Fukushima Daiichi plant in the town of Ōkuma in Futaba county. (See map page vii.)

Ninety-five percent of the personnel in this local regiment are from Fukushima prefecture, including of course the coastal strip known as "Hamadōri".

"Prepare to dispatch the fire engine!"

This unheard-of order came three hours after the earthquake, on the evening of March eleventh.

"The fire engine?"

"What do they want with the fire engine?"

Every JGSDF base is normally equipped with a fire engine. Primarily intended to deal with fires on base, they are occasionally sent to assist at local fires. But this was the first time they'd ever been told to provide a fire engine for disaster relief.

The officers were puzzled at the order.

Even at this stage, before the accident at FDI had become the worst nuclear disaster in history, Site Superintendent Yoshida's plan to use fire engines to cool the reactor had gone into action in the shape of a request for the dispatch of the fire engine from Camp Kōriyama. Generator trucks would also be required, said the request.

Whenever a large earthquake occurs, JGSDF bases are automatically put on immediate Emergency Condition Level Three.

The definition of Emergency Condition Level Three in the Self Defense Force regulations on disaster relief operations states that all personnel are automatically required to report to their posts if an earthquake of local intensity Level 6+ or more occurs in the area for which the unit is responsible.

Since the earthquake at 14:46 and the subsequent tsunami, they had been hastily preparing to assist in relief operations when Yoshida's request for their fire engine reached Camp Kōriyama.

The command was immediately passed on to forty-six-year-old Sergeant Major Hidekatsu Watanabe of the fire-fighting squad under the control of the artillery regiment's command company.

Watanabe knew, of course, that this meant deployment at the nuclear plant. That was something that helped him resign himself to the task.

With a gentle light in his eyes and a manly figure hammered into shape by his job in the military, Watanabe recalled the demanding mission he had been assigned more than a year ago.

"There was another fire engine at JGSDF Camp Fukushima, so we were to rendezvous with them before heading for FDI," he recalled.

After completing their preparations, he and his twelve subordinates waited. The official order came at 23:00. First, six of the men departed directly for FDI in the generator vehicle. Watanabe and the others headed for the Fukushima base to meet the other fire engine and arrive at FDI together.

Watanabe was born at Konan, south of Lake Inawashiro. (See map page vii.) He had a daughter in senior high school. Before setting off, he briefly e-mailed her and his wife.

To his wife he wrote: *Just off to the Fukushima power plant. Could take a few days. Take care of everything.*

To his daughter: *I'm off on a trip. Take care of grandma if anything happens. If you don't hear from me, it means I'm OK. "No news is good news."*

They replied respectively: "RUOK?" and "Hang in there, Dad"

When they were called out to a large relief operation, the soldiers never knew when they'd be able to get back home. This was something inevitable for anyone who signed up for the forces, and his family accepted it.

But since he was heading for a nuclear power station, it held rather more significance than any of his previous disaster relief operations. It wouldn't be surprising if his family were worried about the possibility of radiation. Nor was it surprising that his own thoughts too were different from those on his previous disaster relief operations.

Unaware that the situation at FDI was growing steadily more critical, Watanabe and his six subordinates from Camp Kōriyama, having joined the five from the Fukushima fire-fighting squad, got on the road for FDI, by which time it was already 02:30 on the morning of March twelfth.

Of course there was no way that any of them could have had any idea that their two fire engines were about to play a critical role in cooling the reactors.

In the darkness, they drove east on Route 114. The road was fissured and bumpy, with landslides in some sections, and was occasionally impassable. When that happened, they had to find a detour. Watanabe remembers encountering five or six of them.

As they gradually drew nearer their target, they passed evacuating civilians travelling in the opposite direction.

As the darkness gradually lightened into dawn, they found themselves rolling toward the misty, grey light of the Pacific Ocean.

"Almost dawn," thought Watanabe, and wondered how long they'd been driving. Then he saw a sight that he'd never seen before. The rising sun. A real red rising sun.

"I'd often seen sunsets, but I'd never seen the sun so red in the morning. It was a first. It was really beautiful. And it was rising in precisely the direction we were going. We'd no idea about the casualties there had been in the earthquake and tsunami, and it felt just as if the sun had come out to greet us."

For Watanabe, it was an unforgettable moment.

Soon the main gate of their goal, the FDI plant, appeared. The clock had just passed 07:00.

The stillness wrapped them, and gave no sign of the turmoil within the grounds that would soon shake the whole country.

"Ground Self-Defense Force reporting! Delivering fire engines as requested."

"Wait a moment. I'll get back to you, right away."

Soon one of the TEPCO staff appeared to guide them. "Officer! Boy, are we glad to see you!"

Both Watanabe and the guide were from Fukushima, and once they'd finished their greetings in the musical intonation peculiar to the local dialect, Watanabe got down to business. "We're ready for anything. Tell us what you want us to do."

The TECPO guide told them that they needed help with cooling the reactors, supplying water to the ERC and a mountain of other jobs. But then, Watanabe and his men were held up. Unfortunately, their arrival had coincided with that of the helicopter carrying Prime Minister Kan. They were to waste the next precious hour and a half there at the gate.

Injection

Day 2—March 12 08:30

"SDF reporting. Fire-fighting squad of seven men from Camp Kōriyama."

"Same here. Five men from Camp Fukushima."

It wasn't until after eight thirty, after Kan and his retinue had left, that Sergeant-Major Watanabe and his eleven soldiers finally entered the quakeproof building (QPB). The first floor was bustling with people in Tyvek suits and in the blue TEPCO overalls. There were dozens of them.

"Thank you very much for coming. If you'll come this way we'll explain the job that needs to be done."

Watanabe and his men were led into a small room on the right, where the work was explained to them. One of the management staff came down from the ERC on the second floor to welcome them, and from then on Watanabe and his group were addressed simply as 'Officer.'

Watanabe had a surprise when he mentioned that they had brought food and equipment in their vehicle and would like to go and get them.

"You can't go outside. It's contaminated out there, and no-one is allowed to go out alone anyway," he was told. Going in and out would bring the contamination inside the building, they said, so Watanabe and his crews were not allowed to return to their vehicles. It was an unpleasant way to find out that they'd arrived in the middle of a contaminated area.

Still in their JGSDF camouflage uniforms, they went up to the second floor. Watanabe remembers the looks of shock that they received on entering the ERC.

"Huh? What are the military doing here?" they seemed to ask. It was still the morning after the earthquake, and the uniforms must have impressed the gravity of the situation on the people in the ERC, the command post on the frontline. Greetings began to fly from all corners of the ERC. "Thanks for coming. Good to see you guys." They were friendly, welcoming greetings, unlike the standard format phrases of polite Japanese. For some, the soldiers may even have brought hope that now there was a way out of the crisis.

On returning to the first floor, Watanabe and his men learned how to put on a Tyvek suit. "Put this on. Here are the gloves. That makes a set."

Watanabe realized that their work was going to be even harder wearing these suits to protect them against radioactive contamination. The Tyvek suits don't protect against radiation, only against direct contact, minimizing contamination with radioactive material.

"We'd like you to work on injecting water and cooling Unit 1. TEPCO people will explain the procedure to you when you get to the reactor building. Just follow their instructions. I'll lead you down there, so please follow me in the fire engines."

Without time for a break, Watanabe and his team started on their relief work at 09:00. Their first task was to inject water into Unit 1. (See map page x.)

"I put on the protective mask and then the yellow suit to block radiation, and left the building. Looking down toward the sea, the wreckage was amazing. There were places where the road was impassable, so we cleared away some of the debris and worked our way toward Unit 1. There were cars turned upside down, crushed, or stood on end. One of the TEPCO people told us there had been so much wreckage covering the fire cistern that they couldn't get at the water and had had to hunt for another one. There was a huge oil tank blocking one of the roads, so we couldn't get through that way. When we eventually made our way across the reactor level, we did as we'd been ordered and linked up our fire engine to the one from Fukushima, and then to TEPCO's own fire engine so we could start injecting water.

"The fire engine from Fukushima was set up to draw water from the cistern on the Unit 4 side and pump it through a hose into the tank on the engine from Kōriyama. The Kōriyama vehicle then pumped the water through another hose into the tank on the TEPCO vehicle, which was rigged up to inject water into Unit 1. Injecting water was the only way to cool the reactor, and we did it using what I suppose you could call a 'bucket chain' of three fire engines."

Needless to say, the pipeline *inside* the reactor building was the one set up, at the risk of their lives, by Ōtomo, Hirano and the others from the control room.

"With the masks on, we couldn't hear each other even if we shouted. So we did everything with hand signals. The TEPCO masks had great visibility and were light and easy to breathe in, much better than the military ones we normally used."

The soldiers were able to express everything with hand signals. For instance, raising your arm while doing a thumbs-up meant raise the pressure.

With gestures for 'Lift the hose,' 'Spray,' 'Raise the pressure,' and the like, Watanabe and his team could do everything.

Starting at nine in the morning they worked continuously until about two in the afternoon of March 12.

Watanabe and his men weren't allowed to go back for the food they'd brought with them. In turns, they went up to the second floor and took their meals there instead. The mood in the ERC was tense.

"There were people eating crammed right up against the screen for video conferencing, and around them, as well as in the corridors and stairways, exhausted people lay asleep. The sight of them slumped, made quite an impression on me. They looked really worn out, as if they'd just crumpled on the floor, in their bluish TEPCO overalls, with nothing over or under them. When we came in from our work outside, we put our outer clothes into a bag and handed them over to the TEPCO people. In the lobby we were scanned for radiation and if we were clean, we could go upstairs. Inside the building, we'd change back into our SDF overalls, and when it was time to go out again, we'd change into new Tyvek suits from TEPCO and off we'd go again. By two o'clock we'd repeated that three or four times."

They were walking a narrow line between life and death.

"At the time we didn't realize how dangerous it really was, but when we took the radiation meters they'd supplied us with to the window, we could see the readings rise. I don't know what the units were, but say the figure was a hundred at the middle of the room, it would rise to a hundred and eighty near the windows. It made us wonder what was going on outside. Sometimes the reading even went into four figures, you know. There were times when someone would notice: 'Hey, it's gone up two or three hundred!' They even warned us to keep away from the windows. Naturally, they cautioned us again whenever we went outside, so we kept our masks and suits tightly sealed, not a crack open. You know, we even used packing tape. We wanted to make sure no air got in, so we got dressed very carefully. We understood that our work providing water would help cool the reactor and might help avoid disaster. It might take two weeks, perhaps three, but the operation would carry on, we thought."

The soldiers also helped with a wide range of other work. Not only did they deliver the fire engines, the most urgently required item, but they then stayed to clear the wreckage and generally assist in the vital task of injecting the first of the water into the reactors.

Back into the lion's den

Action!

Day 2—March 12 08:03

"Aim to start the vent at nine o'clock," announced Yoshida as soon as he arrived back in the ERC at 08:03, after his meeting with the PM and his party.

An hour to go till the vent! At last the time was set. Ōtomo and his incursion squad had prepared their equipment and were endlessly rehearsing the process in their minds.

Even though they hadn't slept a wink all night, none of them felt in the least sleepy. Driven by working on the edge, the control room personnel seemed to have lost the ability to sense their own exhaustion. It must have been due to adrenalin.

Besides the equipment they'd had sent over from the depot in the quakeproof building, they had also managed to collect equipment that lay stashed away in the service building: fireproof suits, SCBAs, APDs (Alert Personal Dosimeters) which gave audible warnings, Geiger counters and full-face masks. Gradually they assembled the things they'd need and rehearsed in their minds the actions they'd have to perform inside the reactor building.

If they were going to go into highly radioactive areas, it was essential that they kept the time spent there as short as possible. From the way the radiation was rising, it seemed very probable that the reactor core was already damaged.

To minimize the time spent there, it was vital to visualize the interior of the building and mentally run through the locations of the valves and the various tasks they'd need to perform. As they waited, they sat with their eyes closed and theirs minds churning.

At 06:50 they received the official command from METI minister Kaieda to execute the vent. Now they simply had to wait for confirmation that the local populace had been evacuated.

At 09:02, confirmation arrived that the delayed evacuation of part of Ōkuma was now complete, and two minutes later, the order was given at the ERC.

"Carry out the vent at Unit 1."

Izawa took the call and, with a grim look, passed it on: "Orders from the ERC. Carry out the vent."

"*Ryōkai!*" responded Ōtomo and Ōigawa, who were already dressed in their heavy gear and waiting to go. On top of their Tyvek suits they were wearing armor-like silver fireproof suits, with air tanks on their backs. The heavy equipment made them look very like astronauts about to go on a spacewalk.

Regulations permitted cumulative exposure up to one hundred milliSieverts (mSv) in emergencies, so the APDs they wore were set to warn them when they had been subjected to a total of eighty mSv. They were also supplied with box-shaped portable ionization chamber survey meters, which weighed a full kilogram, to measure the radiation around them as they advanced.

However, in order not to use up their air, they didn't use their tanks until the last moment. On Izawa's signal, they all turned on the last switch on their scubas. The air tanks would last fifteen to twenty minutes during the exercise of normal work, so they had to finish everything within that time.

The pair left the control room without fanfare.

"Oh, God, I hope they get back safely," prayed Izawa. If the core were already damaged, how far had it deteriorated, he wondered. It was impossible to tell. Once they'd seen the two off, there was nothing that those in the control room could do but pray for their safety.

The control room was sunk in silence. No one said a word. They just had to hope that Ōtomo and Ōigawa would fulfill their mission and return safely. That's all they could think about.

The valves

Day 2—March 12 09:05

Ōtomo and Ōigawa walked east down the corridor in the service building where the control room stood, and descended the stairs. At the bottom of the stairs, the two came to the wide passage known as 'The Pine Corridor' that led from the service building to the turbine building and the reactor building. It wasn't so far from there to the double doors at the south entrance to the reactor building. Nevertheless, it was a two-hundred-meter walk from the control room.

For Ōtomo, it was his third visit since the emergency.

He knew from the continually increasing radioactivity that theoretically there was a strong possibility that the core had been damaged. Even though he was just the same person as on earlier incursions, the equipment he'd brought with him this time was completely different.

Nothing told the story of the increased severity of the situation better than the protective gear that enveloped him. Amid the stifling tension, the two of them entered the reactor building by the south-side double doors.

First they climbed the stairs to the second floor. After a short walk, they shone their flashlights above them and in the glow, out of the darkness loomed part of the wall of the huge containment vessel. The vessel was shaped like a laboratory flask, wide at the bottom and narrow at the top. It was thirty-two meters tall but fitted neatly inside the five-story reactor building. At its widest, the containment vessel measured eighteen meters in diameter. (See diagram page ix.)

However, even as they approached the enormous containment vessel it looked like no more than a concrete wall. If this wall were ever breached, the operators' battle would end in defeat. At a minimum, they had to prevent the spread of radioactivity.

It wasn't only their homeland of Fukushima that was at stake; the whole of Japan might never recover. That was something they had to avoid at all costs.

From the second floor of the reactor building, the two of them climbed the stairs beside the heat exchanger. Their only light in the pitch dark came from their handheld flashlights. Carefully illuminating the steps as they climbed, they could just make out the walkway before them.

There was a ladder up ahead. Once they'd climbed that, the valve they were looking for would be one more level above them. For safety, the ladder was enclosed with railings like a fire escape, but with air-tanks on their backs, the metal bars got in their way. It was like climbing inside a metal cage, so they climbed carefully, trying to avoid banging their tanks on the bars. The more-experienced Ōtomo knew these ladders well. Everything went as he'd envisioned it earlier.

"At the top of the ladder, there is a cramped landing, just a metal plate to stand on, and a metal walkway leading to each side. If you go left from there, there is a series of metal steps, and at the top you'll find the valve."

The metal grating walkway was only shoulder-width, forty or fifty centimeters at most. Bending forward, the two of them moved on. Thank goodness there was a railing; even in the pitch black there was no worry that they'd fall. Nevertheless, in their heavy gear, with flashlights in hand, shuffling along the narrow walkway was awkward work.

Ōigawa was in the lead. He carried the ion chamber survey meter to detect radiation, which must have made things all the more difficult.

Ōtomo carried a note with the valve identification number on it. They repeated that number in their heads as they walked. Neither of them realized they were panting. The valve was just up those steps there.

Here we are! they both thought, as they arrived at the bottom of the steps. "There it is!" yelled Ōigawa. They couldn't hear each other in the full-face masks unless they shouted, but his voice reached Ōtomo at the bottom of the steps. It was the valve they wanted. Ōtomo could hear Ōigawa read out the number.

There was no mistake.

"That's the one. No mistake," Ōtomo responded.

"Opening it now," announced Ōigawa as he tried to engage the latch with the gear wheel beside the valve. They had to get it open as soon as they could.

"The latch wouldn't fit into the gear wheel. It took me quite a few tries to get it to fit. But eventually I was able to start turning the handwheel to open the valve," Ōigawa recalls. The wheel itself was only about twenty centimeters across and really stiff. Twenty seconds passed, and thirty.

Normally this would be opened by an electric motor, but he was doing it by hand, in the dark. It was much heavier and stiffer than he'd imagined beforehand.

"Come on, open up!" he begged, and he felt it start to give. It moved! With no time to enjoy his success, he turned the handle for all he was worth.

The display didn't show the valve fully open. Twenty-five percent open, it read. How many times had he turned the wheel to get it that far?

The valve opening gauge beside the valve was marked at five-point intervals. As Ōigawa labored, the needle on the gauge moved slowly across: Five percent, ten percent, fifteen . . . From out of the darkness, Ōtomo's flashlight illuminated its progress.

They had both completely lost track of time. It seemed to have taken forever, but it was also just a moment.

"If we can't do this, we can't save the containment vessel," thought Ōtomo. Veteran that he was, he could think of nothing but saving the containment vessel, which also amounted to saving the reactor.

Without a doubt, if they failed to save the containment vessel, their own lives, their families, perhaps Japan itself, were all done for. But they had no time to think about things like that. The only thing on their minds was saving the containment vessel.

"Come on! We're in a hurry!" he begged.

After about a minute, the needle reached twenty-five percent.

"Check the gauge, would you?" Ōigawa asked his partner. They switched places on the cramped steps. Ōtomo took a look. He could see that the needle indicated twenty-five percent.

"OK!" he cheered as he raised his arms in joy. Not the usual *Ryōkai* or *Daijōbu*! (the Japanese word for OK). The English "OK!" was what shot from his mouth.

The next thing was to get out of there as quickly as they could. The best way to limit radiation exposure was to spend as little time there as possible. They also needed to let the control room know immediately that the valve was now open. But there was no way to communicate except to return and tell them directly.

The SCBA air tanks would last only twenty minutes or so. Their target time for the operation had been set at fifteen minutes and the air tanks had been in use since they left the control room. They had successfully opened the valve, but before they left there was one more thing to do. Ōigawa told his side of the story.

"Since we'd come this far into the reactor building we had a look at the pressures in the containment vessel and the reactor vessel. We had a look at the instruments in the rack there and checked the pressures. It occurred to me that we could use the readings from here to check the accuracy of the readings they'd taken in the control room by connecting batteries to the instruments. I remember looking at the figures and thinking, *What? As high as that?*"

Even though they had to be back in the control room before their air ran out, they took the opportunity on their way back to take pressure readings to calibrate the instruments in the control room!

Ōigawa took the lead again. As he put his hand on the double doors to exit the building, Ōtomo felt a wave of relief.

That zone beyond the double doors was a kind of underworld. Leaving it was like returning to the land of the living.

Mission accomplished! thought Ōtomo, as they walked back to the control room.

At 9:15, the metal door to the control room opened, and there stood the figures of Ōtomo and Ōigawa.

"Hooray!"

"Good job!"

"Welcome back!"

"You made it!"

There must have been more than thirty people in the control room at the time. On the Unit 2 side, the operators were out of the room, trying to find out if the RCIC (which cools the reactor core) was working. Outdoors, people were refueling the fire pump, which had run out of diesel, while others were loading batteries to be used to operate instruments. There was all kind of work under way.

Even with all that going on, there were always at least thirty people in the control room. So when the two came back, there was a clamor of voices from their colleagues hidden in the darkness.

"While they were gone, the control room was really quiet. Not a word from anybody, just silence. Until they got back, we didn't know whether the operation had been successful, or even if they were OK. There was no way to contact them while they were out there. We just had to sit and wait."

Shift supervisor Izawa grimly controlled his impatience.

"It seemed a really long time. In fact, they left at 09:04 and came back at 09:15, so it was only eleven minutes, but it felt like thirty minutes to an hour.

"The control room has a thick metal door, so we didn't hear anything of their footsteps coming down the hallway. The door just suddenly creaked open, and there they were."

Ōigawa traipsed in, followed by Ōtomo, both of them still in all their heavy gear. Everyone in the control room leapt to their feet.

As soon as they had removed their masks, Ōigawa and Ōtomo swung their air tanks off their backs and gasped "It's open!"

"*Yosh!* Good job!" replied Izawa.

The two of them were drenched with sweat, and their faces were flushed with the heat and the strain.

But the valve was open. "They did it!" thought Izawa as he gazed at their rosy faces. Then he immediately phoned the ERC.

"We've opened the valve on the second floor of the reactor. I'll send the second party now."

"Ryōkai!"

The voice of the power generation team manager who'd answered the phone positively bounced. He asked to speak to Ōtomo directly, and cried "Well done, Ōtomo. Great job!

Then they told Izawa the pressure figures for the reactor and the containment vessel that they'd read off the instrument rack inside the reactor building. They corresponded with the high figures recorded in the control room, which meant they needed to finish the vent as soon as possible.

The second party consisted of fifty-one-year-old Hideyoshi Endō and fifty-two-year-old Kazuo Konno. With help from their colleagues they donned the last pieces of their protective gear and heaved their air tanks onto their backs. Once they'd fastened their masks they were ready to go.

"Squad 2. Off you go! We're counting on you."

On Izawa's command, the pair left the control room.

Off the scale!

Day 2—March 12 09:30

The location of the valve that the second party was to open was very different.

The valve that Ōtomo and Ōigawa had opened was on the outside of the concrete wall of the containment vessel. Radiation from the reactor core was blocked by the concrete, so levels were reduced there. The second party's valve was high up above the torus in the suppression chamber downstairs from the reactor, where there was the ceiling, but no concrete wall. Without that concrete wall, there was much less protection against radiation. How much difference it would make to the radiation levels there, nobody really knew. They just had to go and see.

When they returned, the amount of radiation Ōtomo and Ōigawa had been exposed to was calculated at twenty-five and twenty mSv (milliSieverts) respectively.

And they had been subjected to that much in a very short time. If that's how intense the radiation was even outside the concrete wall, the shift supervisor, Izawa, was afraid that the next party, Konno and Endō, might not make it back to the control room.

The minds of these nuclear power veterans were steeped in the potential dangers of radiation. If exposed to intense radiation, human cells would be destroyed, leading to a horrible death. In the 1999 criticality accident at the JCO (Japan nuclear fuel Conversion Office) plant at Tōkaimura in Ibaraki prefecture, workers were exposed to extremely high levels of radiation resulting in severe cellular damage throughout their bodies, leading to gruesome deaths for two of them, an occurrence that the veterans at FDI could never put out of their minds.

The second team went out through the metal door and down the corridor, entering the reactor building by the same double doors as the first team. Endō carried the ion chamber survey meter.

"The double doors on the south side are the kind that have to be unlatched with a clunk before they'll open. It was my first time inside Unit 1 since the earthquake and I'd heard that the radiation levels were high, up around five hundred," commented Endō.

"*Yosh!*" he barked as he opened the inner doors. "Here goes!"

"We opened the outer doors and went inside, and, with our

eyes on the meter, clunked the inner doors open. I guess I yelled '*Yosh!*' like that to fire myself up. Once we were inside, the needle on the meter was at five or six hundred."

Endō's "battle cry" must have helped him to brace himself. The inside of the dark building, lit up by their flashlights, was enveloped in whitish haze.

"We didn't know if that white haze was steam or dust. We came in from the south side and followed the south-side corridor and then turned north on the west-side corridor toward the northwest corner, where we went downstairs."

It goes without saying that the radiation levels varied from place to place. When they reached the northwest corner, the needle had dropped to around two hundred, but on the way there they had passed areas where it had read nine hundred.

Time was limited, and as they neared their objective, they unconsciously started to jog.

"We'd heard beforehand that the north side was less radioactive, and when we got there we found that for some reason it was true. The entrance to the torus room, where the donut-shaped suppression chamber is located, is on a slightly lower level, sunk into the floor, and from there we finally entered."

Endō and Konno nodded to each other, and opened the door. They'd no idea what they'd find on the other side.

"Once we were inside we could hear a hammering noise. It was probably the noise of reactor exhaust steam bubbling into the torus, but it really echoed around. Outside the door the meter had read six hundred, but once we opened the door it went up to nine hundred. The needle was jumping about a bit so sometimes it went to a thousand, sometimes nine hundred. You could change the scale on the meter to cover all ranges from zero to a thousand, but it was almost to its limit. At least it was still in the measurable range, I thought, and so we went on."

There's no going back now. The two carried on. Eventually they climbed the steps up the outside of the toroidal suppression chamber itself and onto the meter-wide catwalk that ran around it.

The needle was still at around nine hundred.

"As long as it's still on the scale, let's keep going."

Endō was getting desperate. The extreme levels of radiation threatened their very lives, but there was no choice but to go on.

"We turned left onto the catwalk, going clockwise around to our target. The target valve was a hundred and eighty degrees around, on the far side. We had to go halfway around from the north side, but on the way there was what we called the ninety-degree hatch. This was an opening for maintenance, and when we got there the needle hit the end of the scale."

The needle of Endō's ion chamber survey meter, which could measure up to a thousand, was pressed hard against the pin, motionless. It didn't waver or bounce back.

This meant that they were in the midst of unimaginable radiation.

They couldn't go on.

Feelings of futility welled within him. But beyond here the radiation levels would undoubtedly be even higher. That way led only to a tragic end.

Endō decided to turn back. They had to work out a new plan.

But Konno, five meters behind him, was unaware of the danger. Endō spun around and waved at him to stop.

"I waved the meter at him. *Look, look at this,* I pointed, trying to explain to him. The actual figures, or whether he could even read them, didn't matter. Just that the needle was off the scale. *It's too dangerous. We can't go any further,* was all I wanted to tell him. We had to get out of there as quickly as possible, so I pushed past Konno, grabbed his arm and dragged him backwards."

Konno understood, of course, that the radiation level had shot up. It was a shock, but the thought uppermost in his mind was that they wouldn't be able to complete the vent.

Even though they had to get out of there as quickly as possible, Konno froze. He was suddenly paralyzed.

Endō just heaved him along regardless. On the way, he lost his grip, and when he at last reached the double doors, he turned, only to find that Konno was no longer with him.

"As I went to open the inside door, I looked around and saw that Konno wasn't there. I was really surprised and, for a moment, concerned. But before I could make up my mind what to do, I saw him appear around the corner about ten meters away, heading towards me, so I waved for him to hurry."

Until they turned back, Konno hadn't been looking at the

readings on the meter, so it was a huge shock to suddenly learn they were giving up.

"My legs wouldn't move! I was enervated. I just felt too heavy to carry on," Konno explained laconically.

Neither of them had noticed the APD alarms that they'd stuffed into their pockets. Under their full-face masks, the racket from the torus had completely drowned out the tiny *pip-pip-pip* of the alarms.

When the two of them got back to the control room they were so utterly exhausted that people gathered around to make sure they were all right.

"It was no good, . . ." sighed Endō, as he took off his gear.

"The radiation was too high. It was no good. The meter was off the scale," he continued, squeezing out the words.

The meter was off the scale! That was what they'd been afraid of. There was already too much radiation in the building for anyone to go inside. That was the hard-boiled reality that Endō's brief words implied.

How could they run the vent now? What other method could they devise? Izawa and his team were up against a new situation.

"It was so hot. The mask kept fogging up so I couldn't see."

As they removed their equipment they described the operation in the torus room a few words at a time. It had obviously been far tougher than any of them had expected.

"When we checked their exposure meters we found they read eighty-something and ninety-something. That was a whole lot worse than the first party," commented Izawa. The precise figures were eighty-nine mSv for Endō and ninety-five mSv for Konno. In one short burst, they had been exposed to four times as much radiation as Ōtomo and Ōigawa, who had gone only a little earlier.

By law, the limit for exposure is set at one hundred mSv. With the exposure they had undergone, there was no choice but to order them out of danger. Izawa soon told both of them to evacuate to the ERC building.

"The legal limit for cumulative exposure while dealing with an accident is one hundred mSv, and the level in the control room was slowly rising, so it would be dangerous for them to hang around. So I ordered them to take refuge in the QPB. They simply had to get out of the control room," said Izawa.

When Konno saw what the radiation levels inside the reactor building had been, and what the figures for their exposure were, he accepted for the first time that they'd made the correct decision in turning back.

Endō, who had grabbed Konno's arm and desperately dragged him back, was already thinking hard about the next plan of attack.

"At the time, I'd realized we had no choice but to turn back. Before noon we were evacuated to the ERC. But at the time all I could think about was what to do next. What options did we have left? It wasn't quite a test flight, but we'd gone and taken a look, and found out what the situation was. What we did next was no longer a matter for us in the control room to decide. Now it was up to the ERC."

At the ERC, Endō and Konno continued to pursue alternative methods. However, even in the ERC, their cumulative exposure continued to mount and they became the first personnel at the Fukushima Daiichi plant to exceed the one hundred mSv limit. On March thirteenth they were evacuated to the Offsite Center. Yoshida ordered them to see the doctor.

"Because we were contaminated, they scanned us when we arrived at the Offsite Center. It was as if we were aliens from outer space," laughed Endō.

"At the main entrance to the Offsite Center there was a side door, and once we'd got inside, we found a decontamination space with a shower. Still no heating or lights, of course, not even warm water. It was March, so it was still freezing outside. Anyway, we washed off the contamination while we shook with the cold."

But the decontamination wasn't over.

"We were taking our cold water showers practically outdoors, and kept scrubbing away, but however many times they scanned us, they said it was still no good. We scrubbed and scrubbed, and I think was about the fifth time, at last they said we were OK. Then we had all kinds of creams plastered on. They took all our belongings away. Our watches and phones were contaminated, they said, so they took them away. They stripped us completely naked, and we didn't even have any overalls, so they gave us some prefectural staff uniforms. So we dressed up in those prefectural staff outfits and stayed in the Offsite Center."

The taxing preparations for the vent had been a battle not only against the rising radiation figures, but also a struggle against fear. It had turned into an integrated operation bound together by the technicians' theory and practical experience.

Don't leave!

Civilian evacuation

Day 2—March 12 Dawn

At dawn on March 12, the tension at Tomioka's Disaster Response Headquarters (DRHQ) in *Manabi no Mori* was rising. (See map page vii.)

Makoto Kamino, aged forty-two, head of the Tomioka office of the local newspaper, *Fukushima Minpō*, had returned to the Disaster Response Headquarters on the second floor of the arts center.

"What's a vent?" he asked. The foreign word was totally unfamiliar (and, when squeezed into the Japanese syllabary, pronounced *bento*). TEPCO had announced that there was going to be one and that they were getting ready to carry it out. The DRHQ was in even more of an uproar now that they had been told to evacuate all the civilians within ten kilometers of the plant before the operation was carried out.

But what is a vent? thought Kamino. *What happens if you do one? On the other hand, what happens if you don't?* Kamino wasn't alone. Hardly anyone in the building knew what the word really meant. Kamino decided to question the PR officer from Fukushima Daini nuclear power plant who was holed up in the DRHQ office about this and other basic points.

"I'd honestly never heard the word *vent* before. I hadn't a clue what it meant. There can't have been more than a handful of people in the Tomioka DRHQ who knew what it meant," Kamino declared. But as soon as he heard the explanation he understood.

"To put it simply, it means letting the gas out. I understood it to mean that some air would be released but it would be only slightly radioactive."

The problem was safety. That was everyone's concern. The PR officer from Fukushima Daini nuclear power plant explained "It's not something that will have a really critical effect," and continued "depending on the wind direction . . ." At which everyone from the Mayor on down looked outside to the large balcony of the Disaster Response Headquarters where the town flag rippled on its pole. It wasn't yet 06:00 in the morning. The night was not yet over. The town flag fluttered, pointing east toward the sea.

"TEPCO was obliged to explain to the Tomioka town officials what was going on, and I was there for that meeting. The gist of it was that the vent would release some air from inside, but it wouldn't be *that* radioactive. The area was still in a blackout, and the DRHQ had a couple of generators out on the balcony, so it was pretty noisy at the meeting. One of the town officials asked about the wind direction and everyone turned to look at the flag outside. I remember we were all somewhat relieved to see it was pointing out to sea."

At six fifty in the morning, the municipal public address system broadcast the order to evacuate.

At the time, two more of the newspaper's staff were present in the DRHQ besides Kamino. The previous evening, a reporter and a photographer from head office had come to support him. He had sent them to cover the press conference at Ōkuma town hall and they had now come back.

Apparently, only two news agencies had attended that press conference – NHK (the national broadcasting agency) and their own *Fukushima Minpō*.

At the moment, the photographer was in his car, catching up on some sleep. Kamino guessed that once the evacuation got under way, the roads would be clogged, so he went out to the car and knocked on the window.

Waking the photographer, he told him, "They've just broadcast an evacuation order. Could you go on ahead to Kawauchi? I think the traffic will get bad soon." The village of Kawauchi was almost twenty kilometers away among the mountains to the west. They had electric power there. It was vital that his support team move there now and avoid the traffic jams that would inevitably occur once the evacuation got under way.

"I'll stay here, so you two go ahead. You can interview the evacuees in Kawauchi and send your report to head office. "

The two set off immediately.

But the road to Kawauchi was already lined with cars like beads on a rosary. People had reacted to the evacuation announcement promptly, so they made little progress. The photos that later appeared in the *Fukushima Minpō* newspaper were of scenes of the evacuation on the road to Kawauchi.

A little after two in the afternoon at the DRHQ in Tomioka, the atmosphere suddenly changed. Among the scrolling bulletins at the bottom of the TV screen, there was an item saying that cesium had been detected in the area of FDI.

"Cesium? Damn it! That's serious!" Mayor Endō murmured to himself, but Kamino overheard. Cesium (strictly speaking, the isotope Cs-137) is one of the elements created inside nuclear reactors. That this had been detected indicated that a substance that had been produced inside a reactor had escaped into the outside world. It meant that radioactive contamination had become a reality.

"Now we're screwed!" Kamino heard the mayor mutter to himself, and realized how bad the situation really was. There were still fifty or sixty people in the Tomioka DRHQ at the time. Immediately afterwards, the mayor faced the whole assembly and gave them their instructions.

"Listen, everyone!" he started. "We've heard that cesium has been detected. I will remain here with a few core staff, using protective gear, to keep things running, but I want the rest of you to evacuate immediately."

The DRHQ itself was evacuating! If all but a few senior staff were to evacuate, the functions of the Disaster Response Headquarters would effectively be lost. The situation couldn't be much more serious than this.

The possible horrors of a nuclear accident welled up afresh in Kamino's mind.

"Only the most senior staff were to remain; the mayor, the head of security and a few other department heads. The fire brigade, after receiving orders from the mayor, then got further instructions from the Fire Chief and commenced their evacuation. I decided that, having followed the situation this far, I'd better go to Kawauchi too. Even though cesium had been detected, I only imagined that I'd be leaving Tomioka for two or three days. I set off in my own car. There was hardly anyone left in Tomioka, so there were no more traffic jams, and I sailed through the deserted town on my way to Kawauchi."

It must have been about ten minutes later, before he'd even left the town limits, that Kamino noticed a large bus coming the other way. As it came closer, he saw that the passengers were all dressed in protective clothing – white Tyvek suits. He couldn't tell if they were from TEPCO or some other organization, but there was no mistake; meeting such a group on a lonely road was a sure indicator of the scale of the radiation accident.

They're on their way to try to control the damage, thought Kamino as the huge bus passed by.

"It's all up to you now, guys!" he muttered. Even before the evacuation from the Tomioka DRHQ had started, town hall staff had gone out on their surveys in protective clothing and had still been wearing them when they reported back to the mayor, so Kamino was already used to figures in white Tyvek suits.

But as he gripped the steering wheel, he got the feeling that the increasingly uninhabited surrounding townships were gradually turning into a dead zone.

Retry

Day 2—March 12 10:00

Executing the vent manually from inside the reactor building would be impossible, they were told. This message from the control room was a shock for those in the ERC.

The jubilation that shortly before had filled the room at the news of the success of the first squad was replaced by oppressive gloom. But under Yoshida's direction they had already started devising an alternative method. They were investigating the possibilities for executing the vent from outside.

The recovery team, who were going flat out in the ERC, had come up with an idea.

"Couldn't we use an air-compressor and inject air to open the pneumatic AO valve?"

Instead of opening it by hand, perhaps they could open the

valve remotely using air pressure. It might not work, but it was worth a try.

First they needed a compressor. The recovery team immediately began a search. There must be one on site somewhere.

They found one – it was two meters long and one meter in height and width. The next problem was whether they could find a connector that would fit properly. Numerous suggestions were raised and tested, one by one, until eventually they had something that they could go ahead and try out for real.

Endō and Konno had reached the ERC at about noon on March 12. They had been exposed to almost one hundred mSv of radiation, so Izawa had ordered them to withdraw to the QPB. Forty-eight-year-old Kazuhiro Yoshida of the operations management department was attached to the power generation team at the time and remembers seeing the expressions of fatigue on the pair's faces as they entered the ERC.

"They were both soaked in sweat and came in looking apologetic for being a nuisance. They looked absolutely worn out so I got up and commended them for their efforts."

Kazuhiro Yoshida was second in command of the D-shift of the team responsible for Units 5 and 6 at FDI, but when he started work at FDI, he'd been posted at Units 1 and 2, and had accumulated more than ten years' experience there.

He was originally from Minami Sōma (about twenty kilometers north of the plant) and had a son in college and a daughter at high school. Though he was off-duty at the time, as soon as the earthquake struck he had left his home in Futaba and come to help, working all night removing wreckage and trying to restore Units 5 and 6. Landslips and the collapse of a power pylon during the earthquake had restricted access around the two northernmost units.

But the continually deteriorating state of Units 1 and 2 concerned him enormously. At the time, he was the only member of the power generation team left in the ERC who had as much experience at Units 1 and 2.

He, more than any of his fellows, felt attached to those reactors and was determined to save them.

"I was brought up on those reactors, so I was really fond of them. I'd worked on them for years, so I really felt I had to look after them, almost like the attachment we have to our children. In the middle of the night, when Unit 1 started getting really bad, I asked them to let me go to the control room, but they told me it was out of the question. *You're responsible for Units 5 and 6,* I was told. So I had to stay and help out with Units 5 and 6."

But when Endō and Konno were evacuated to the ERC, the situation changed. If these two veterans had left the Unit 1 and 2 control room, they must need somebody to stand in for them.

"I'm the only man for the job," thought Kazuhiro Yoshida.

"Is there someone who'll go?"

When the second in command of the power generation team asked for volunteers, Yoshida spoke up immediately.

"I'll go!" he responded. Shift supervisor Izawa, who was battling on in the control room for Units 1 and 2, was one of Yoshida's seniors at high school, which gave them an extra degree of attachment.

His beloved reactors were being defended by his senior, shift supervisor Izawa. For Yoshida, the choice was clear.

"You come, too," he suggested to Yoshihiro Satō, one of his juniors who was standing at his side.

"Yoshihiro and I went to the same high school. He was one year behind me and in the basketball club, while I was in athletics. He was on the Unit 3 and 4 team, so when I suggested he join me in going to Units 1 and 2, he looked really surprised."

In high school, Yoshida had been a good middle distance runner and had placed in the eight hundred meters event in the Fukushima prefecture championships. Satō's basketball team had won the prefecture championships, and he, too, was fast on his feet. After the failed second incursion, the two of them were sent to replace the two shift supervisors from the control room. There might be something they could do; Yoshida could think of nothing else.

The two were on first name terms.

"It was a surprise when Kazuhiro looked at me and said 'You come, too,' but I knew right away he was going to do something about the vent. I was on the Unit 3 and 4 team, and hadn't been into Units 1 and 2 team since a short spell there about twenty-five years before, so I was a bit nervous. But I thought, *if I'm with Kazuhiro I'll be fine,*" Satō recounted.

When they arrived at the control room there was a chorus of welcome. "Are we glad to see you!"

Even simply visiting the control room involved an element of danger now, and that feeling of solidarity between fellow operators must also have contributed to their welcome.

"As I opened the door to the control room, I didn't know what to say."

The weirdness of the situation in the room hit him.

"I'd already heard a bit about what it was like in there so I wasn't exactly surprised, but my first impression was *Wow! It couldn't be much worse than this!* Normally, as operators, we assume that even if the power goes down, we will still have the DC supply, so we assume that, whatever happens, at least the lights will be on. But the lights were out. Even the emergency lights were out. I really thought, *This must be as bad as it gets!* When we arrived there were people gathered around fluorescent tubes rigged up on the desks, and when we walked in they really made us welcome. Personally, I was glad just to have got this far."

Their senior from high school, Izawa, had something different to say. "So you're the suicide squad, are you? I guess you're here because you can run. "

Suicide squad? Run? thought Yoshida, but before he had time to puzzle it out, he found out exactly what Izawa meant.

"I want to give it another try."

They'd already been discussing this very topic in the control room. They had been forced to abandon their first attempt at opening the AO valve when the needle on the radiation detector had gone off the scale, but now they were discussing the possibility of another try.

The idea was that they might be able to open the valve manually from inside the reactor building. This time it would have to be carried out by the third team, Hirano and fifty-year-old Kenji Miyata, who were now steeling themselves to the task.

Hirano's dilemma

Day 2—March 12 14:00

"We need to talk," Izawa summoned his team of veterans to the space on the Unit 1 side of the central work table. They were about to hammer out a plan for a final attempt on the vent.

Kazuhiro Yoshida told me his side of the story.

"I remember that, at this point, Hirano and Miyata had said they would go. I seem to recall they were already partly dressed to go. They were discussing which route to take into the reactor building; this way had so much radiation, that way had so much, how about this way, and that kind of thing. But Hirano said that to be sure of the actual position of the valve, they would have to go and see for themselves. That got people a bit worried. *Wasn't there anyone who knew the layout properly?* they asked."

That was when Kazuhiro spoke up.

"I know the layout. Why not let me go?"

With more than ten years of experience working on the Unit 1 reactor, Kazuhiro Yoshida knew all there was to know about the location of the AO valve. He could see the thing in his mind.

"I can run faster than Hirano, too," he remembered to add. Kazuhiro was eight years younger than Hirano, and had been a middle-distance prizewinner in the prefectural high school athletics contest. He knew he could run. What was more, he'd left the ERC for the control room with his mind set on executing the vent himself.

Kazuhiro spoke laughingly but Hirano was dead serious. He was already well aware that it could be fatal. He couldn't send anyone younger (and hence more vulnerable to radiation) than himself into that place.

"It's my responsibility. I'll do it myself," Hirano announced to all present. The second team had turned back when the radiation went off the scale. He couldn't let the youngsters go in there.

Kazuhiro recalls that there was then some discussion with Hirano. Hirano had looked him straight in the face. "It's too dangerous. Have you any idea how much radiation there is?" he'd asked.

"Hirano told me he couldn't allow me to go. But the man running the show was Izawa. He pointed out that I had more chance of success and tried to persuade Hirano to let me go. But Hirano carried on being stubborn"

Now it was Izawa's turn to be adamant.

"Kazuhiro knows exactly where the valve is, Hirano. We must let him do it."

At last Hirano was brought around.

"I'll go, then," concluded Kazuhiro, and Hirano was obliged to hold his tongue.

"Hirano already had a fireproof suit over his shoulders. The others helped him off with his gear and put it on me. He was still trying to resist, but now it had been decided that I'd go with Satō, there was nothing more he could say," Kazuhiro Yoshida explained.

So Izawa had entrusted the 'return match' to his juniors in the athletics and basketball teams.

Satō and Yoshida chatted as they put on their gear.

"I'm going to run. OK?"

"I guessed that much!"

The less time they spent in the radiation, the better. The more time they spent there, the more damage they'd incur. Their solution was to run.

However, as they put on their gear they began to have qualms. With air tanks on their backs, SCBA sets, their full-face masks sealed with tape, and wearing huge rubber boots, they wondered if they would really be able to run at all. For a start, the mouthpiece of the breathing apparatus had two layers, making both speaking and hearing difficult.

The amount of equipment was rather more than they'd anticipated. But now there was nothing left to do but go.

"I was going in to save my beloved reactor, and the time had come, I thought. But all I could think about was our route through the building and how to open the valve. Anyway, we'd keep one eye on the radiation meter and go as far as we could, I thought."

They decided not to take the heavy ion chamber radiation meter this time, just their personal dosimeters (APD) hung around their necks, set to go off when they had counted eighty mSv.

"We already knew from the earlier visits that the radiation on the first floor of the building was seventy to eighty mSv per hour and that it was about a hundred on the north side, so we'd been told to go around the south side because the levels were lower there. If the radiation reached a certain level we'd be over the permissible limits in no time. The problem we foresaw was with the levels we'd find *after* we'd crossed the first floor and gone through the door down into the torus room. We were sure we'd have no trouble getting as far as the door to the torus room. After that we'd just have to run. But if we accumulated a hundred mSv on the way in, we'd inevitably pick up another hundred on the way out, so we'd be crazy not to turn back then. The problem was how much radiation there was, and where. That was what would make or break the operation."

The two slipped out of the control room.

Stop them!

Day 2—March 12 A little later

It was only a moment after the two had steeled themselves and set off for the reactor building when the phone from the ERC rang in the control room.

"There's white smoke coming out of the ventilation stack. Is the control room OK?"

White smoke coming out of the stack? Izawa paled as he took the call. He'd instantly sensed danger.

The ventilation stack is, as its name suggests, a chimney for expelling air from inside the reactor building. If it were simply the exhaust from the air-conditioning it would be no problem. But there remained the possibility that something serious was going on in there. And people were on their way into the building at that very moment.

"Stop them!"

Izawa was surprised at his own vehemence. He meant of, course, the two who had just departed for the reactor building.

The first to react were assistant shift supervisor Katō and his immediate superior, deputy shift supervisor Homma. The moment Izawa bellowed, Homma, who was the nearer to the door, grabbed a flashlight and a mask and dashed out.

"Stop those two!"

By the time Izawa had re-worded his command, Homma was out of the door, pulling on his mask as he raced off with Katō in pursuit. If the incursion team managed to enter the reactor building, it would be too late to stop them.

They didn't know what the problem was. All they knew was that the ERC had called them on the hotline to say that something was going down, and shift supervisor Izawa had yelled "Stop them!"

There was no doubt it was an emergency. That was why Homma had dashed out of the control room.

Homma reminisced, "The urgency in Izawa's voice was incredible. As soon as he took the call from the ERC he hollered 'Stop them!' so we knew something had happened and they had to be stopped. We didn't know what the reason for stopping them was, though. Just that they had to be stopped. They'd left only a few minutes before, so we should be able to catch up with them, I thought. We set off after them.

Homma had an idea. If he took a short cut through the changing room on the second floor and then cut through the warehouse, he'd be able to catch up with them. Sure enough, as he came out and ran down the stairs he could see their backs ahead of him.

"Stop! Stop!" he roared at the top of his voice, but the sound didn't reach them. Oblivious inside the protection of fireproof suits, breathing apparatus and full-face masks, they hurried on. There was no way they could have heard him, however loud he shouted.

"O-o-o-o-oy! Wait!" he yelled again, still running.

When he finally caught up with the pair, they were fifty meters from the reactor building doors. Kazuhiro Yoshida and Hirano were walking. They'd been held up climbing over a pile of cabinets that had been toppled by the earthquake and tsunami. That was the only reason Homma had been able to catch up.

"Come back!" Homma bawled, grabbing Kazuhiro's shoulder backward. Both of them were wearing air tanks on their backs, it was the only way to get their attention.

Homma, once a member of his school judo club, weighed a hundred kilograms. Imagine a man of that size charging forward and suddenly grabbing your shoulder. Kazuhiro was astonished. He was wearing a full-face mask over his SCBA equipment. He couldn't hear a thing, and wasn't aware of anything until, out of the blue, Homma heaved on his shoulder.

"After grabbing my shoulder, Homma shouted at me 'Come back!' I was startled. I didn't immediately understand what he meant and shouted back, 'What for?' We'd steeled ourselves to it and gotten this far. Then Homma yelled, 'You are ordered to return to the control room'. I remember I angrily snapped back at him that this was no time to be telling me something like that."

If he hadn't been so fired up, Kazuhiro wouldn't have risked life and death making this sortie into the midst of all that radioactive contamination in the first place. That was the only reason he resisted Homma's instructions to turn back.

But Homma and Yoshida were from completely different generations. And Yoshida was the senior.

"Kazuhiro was furious. He bawled me out. But I'd been told by the control room to bring him back, so I pleaded with him: 'Well, at least come back and see what's up. The order comes from the ERC.'"

Homma was beside himself. It was at this moment that Katō managed to catch up with them, and he gestured for Kazuhiro to turn back.

That was how the two were saved from going into the reactor building.

"It sent a shiver down my back, to think what might have happened if they had gone inside the building. Kazuhiro didn't understand what was going on when he was suddenly dragged back, he says. It was a close thing," recalls Izawa.

But what *was* that white smoke after all? It could be that the reactor core had been damaged and the fuel rods exposed, boiling off some water into steam, or it could be that some hydrogen from somewhere had combusted and left a white vapor. At that point Izawa didn't know.

It later became clear that, as a result of the injection of air, the AO valve on Unit 1 had opened and released the pressure from the containment building; in other words, it indicated a successful vent.

Nevertheless, in the control room they were unaware of this, and the operators there were fixated with the conclusion that entering the reactor building was now impossible. The control room was heavy with despair and the bitter taste of doom.

The junior operators

Day 2—March 12 15:00

"Chief, is there really any point in us being here?"

The question from one of the younger operators, addressed to Izawa, came without warning, a little later. He spoke loudly. When the question boomed around the dark room, Izawa and the other shift supervisors were standing at the communal work table in the center of the control room, discussing their next moves.

On the orders of the site superintendent, Masao Yoshida, they had worked on restoring power, on using a compressor to open the vent valve, and on other tasks, but time had gone by and they had heard nothing of the results of their labors.

For the younger operators, it felt as if they were just killing time.

On behalf of a number of the youngsters, one of them had spoken up. Most of them were huddled on the Unit 2 side of the room, where the radiation was the lowest. The question summed up their concerns.

"There's nothing for us to do here. Is there any point in us staying? Couldn't we go back to the ERC and make ourselves useful there? We can come back here once it's been decided what to do, can't we? There must be a better way," he continued. It was a valid point. Visits to the reactor building and all the other jobs where there was a risk of irradiation were carried out by the older men. The younger men had been restricted to reading the instruments, keeping watch for further tsunamis and the like, but there wasn't much of that kind of work now.

Is there really any point in us being here? Exactly! It was a fundamental question for all who remained in the control room.

In the dim light of the glowing fluorescent tubes, Izawa noticed a few of the seated operators nodding unobtrusively to each other.

At the young man's words, all kinds of things ran through Izawa's mind, such as the places he'd grown up in. It was true that there was little work for the younger operators now. But there were still plenty of small jobs that needed doing, and it was quite possible to imagine a situation where they'd still need plenty of manpower.

The silence dragged on.

"If we abandon the control room . . ."

Izawa eventually started to reply. The silence was daunting. They waited for him to continue.

"If we aba, . . . " he repeated, but the words wouldn't come. He was too choked with emotion. "Abandoning the control room means . . . we abandon the plant . . . and the whole region around it." Bit by bit he wrung the words out. "The people who have already evacuated are watching us and praying that we can do something," he continued, choking on his words. "So we can't . . . there's no way we can just throw in the towel here."

Izawa had been brought up here, in the Hamadōri area, and found scenes of his youth whirling in his head. "I beg you." His voice had gradually dropped.

"I won't send any of you into danger. If things get dangerous here, I'll use my authority to have you all evacuated. Until then . . ." He summoned his strength for the conclusion. "I beg you. Stay!" He said no more, but merely bowed his head. His words had been squeezed out one by one.

The operators had nothing to say. As tears welled, Izawa kept his head bowed and retired backward into the gloom.

If he had stayed out in front he might not have been able to control his tears. As shift supervisor, as a man, he couldn't allow his subordinates to see him cry.

Hirano, who had been standing diagonally behind him, stepped forward. Simultaneously, Ōtomo, too, took two or three steps forward. Shielding Izawa from view, they stood in silence with their heads bowed.

Izawa, Hirano and Ōtomo, the three senior officers, stood, bowed in supplication to their subordinate operators. The younger men were speechless.

Hirano recalls his feelings at the time.

"Normally, as the most senior officer there, I should have said something before Izawa, but it all happened so suddenly, I couldn't react in time. By the time I'd got my words together, Izawa had already started to speak. I feel really bad about it, even now. He promised them he wouldn't send them into danger and begged them to stay a little longer. . . ."

"What were you going to say?" I enquired.

"I was going to say that, for young and old alike, there would be situations when we, as TEPCO staff, had to take responsibility, and even, to a degree, make sacrifices in order to protect the people of the area and to protect the nation."

It was the place for heroism. If things continued the way they were going, their hometown would be wiped out. The shift supervisors mustered their courage. What Hirano had wanted to say to the junior operators was about resigning themselves. If he had expressed it himself he would probably have included more anger, he admits.

"Resigning yourself means being prepared to do everything it takes, right to the end. When a nuclear plant gets into this kind of state, you can't get by with half-hearted measures, can you? If worse came to worst, we'd have to contain the damage as best we could, and we operators on the frontline might have to make sacrifices to do what needed to be done. How can I put it? It's an operator's responsibility. . . ."

While he was debating with himself how he could explain it to them, Izawa had spoken up, says Hirano.

"I couldn't get the words right in my head, and while I was still thinking the best way to put it, Izawa stepped up and started speaking. Once he'd finished, there was nothing for me to do but dip my head and hold my tongue."

Izawa had already decided that he would remain to the very end, even if he had to stay there alone.

But he had no intention of making the younger operators die there with him. It was just that while there was work to do, he wanted them to stay.

Out of the silence, Izawa, with his head still bowed, spoke again. "One more thing: Not all of us are operators. There is also a trainee here."

Purely by coincidence, one young man who had been in the control room at the time of the earthquake was still only training to become an operator. That's who Izawa meant.

"He's not an operator yet. I'd like to evacuate him to the ERC. Okay?"

He made sure that they understood, and heads nodded all around. They'd also agreed that they'd remain in the control room.

Two of the operators escorted the trainee to the ERC, but just after they had all seen them on their way, something happened that neither Izawa nor Hirano had anticipated.

Explosion at Unit 1

The fifth floor, gone?

Day 2—March 12 15:36

Izawa and his team were lifted from the ground. It was quite different from the earthquake's aftershocks that had plagued them repeatedly. People fell from their chairs, or were bounced up off the floor, still sitting, while others were simply bowled over. Fluorescent tubes and ventilation louvers crashed down from the ceiling.

"Masks! Get your masks on!" screamed Izawa, as dust danced, casting a white haze throughout the room. The portable generator that had been carried in last night and had gallantly kept a number of lamps on the desks dimly lit, died.

"There was absolutely no warning. Just BOOM! We didn't know what it was. For a moment, I had a feeling there had been a steam explosion in the pressure vessel and that the whole reactor had gone up," said Izawa.

"When the earthquake came there was a kind of process to it; first there was a sort of underground rumbling and then the shaking started, but with this we were suddenly just hammered by this incredible THUMP. I just hung onto the floor," recalled Homma, the deputy shift supervisor.

It was 15:36 on March 12 when the explosion occurred in the reactor building at Unit 1.

"Oh, no!" thought Izawa, as he remembered the three who had just set off for the ERC. He'd told them to call as soon as they got there. Izawa wouldn't allow anyone to do anything outside alone. That was why he'd sent two of the operators to escort the trainee: so that one of them wouldn't have to come back alone.

And the explosion had come before they had reported their safe arrival.

"Find out if those three have reached the ERC, will you?" Izawa ordered the man at the hotline.

"They've arrived!" the man reported back. They'd been scanned and had just climbed the stairs to the ERC when the explosion occurred.

They still didn't know what had exploded.

"At first we didn't know what had happened. We asked the ERC but they didn't know either. In fact the ERC even asked *us,* wondering if perhaps one of our generators had blown up, but we in the control room were blind to the outside world; if the ERC didn't know, then we didn't know either. Something must have happened to the reactor; and it was definitely something big. We were all asking each other what it could be."

Now that Izawa and his team were all wearing masks all the time, simply speaking to each other had become more difficult. Eventually a call came from the ERC.

"Hey, the fifth floor of the reactor building is gone!"

What? The fifth floor, gone? No way! That's impossible! Izawa and his masked team in the dark couldn't believe what they heard from the ERC.

"They said the fifth floor of the reactor building was gone. We discussed what might have happened; it could have been this, it might have been that; no, it couldn't have been that, and the like; but not one of us had imagined beforehand that the fifth floor could just get blown away like that. Even after hearing about it, we were still puzzling over what it meant."

The shock of the explosion had been terrific even in the ERC, four hundred meters away from the reactor building.

"It wasn't so much a noise like an explosion as a feeling, like being punched by the ground. In the corridor to the link that connects to the admin building, the ceiling collapsed with a bang. An earthquake shouldn't cause it to collapse, so we thought perhaps somewhere in the quakeproof building there had been a gas leak or something, and it had blown the ceiling down."

This is what Masaru Sekiya, who was in charge of the radiation meters at the entrance to the QPB, had to say. Seen from the entrance, the air outside seemed to turn grey as something started to rain down.

"The main corridor from the entrance to the QPB leads straight through to a back door that faces toward Unit 1. The door was made of steel, but it had been crumpled by the blast. Together we kicked it back into good enough shape that it could be closed, and then sealed the remaining gaps with packing tape. As you come in the front entrance, there is a connecting corridor on the left that links across to the main administration building, and, just before you reach the link itself, there is an intake vent known as a 'damper' for the air-conditioning. Normally, this draws fresh air in from outside and passes it through a charcoal filter to provide clean air for the QPB, but in this case it had provided a channel for the blast to come in and knock down the ceiling panels in the corridor near the link."

That's how strong the blast was: enough to bring down the ceiling of a corridor in the quakeproof building!

"This meant that the corridor in the QPB was now wide open to the outside air! The ceiling had fallen down all the way along the side corridor from the damper to the link. The connecting link has an upper story, and the ceiling upstairs had fallen down, too; both the first and second floors were completely open to the outside air."

Consequently, of course, the radioactive contamination readings were going up.

"After the blast, the Geiger-Müller survey meter, which reads up to a hundred thousand counts per second, went off the scale. On the inside of the glass at the entrance to the QPB, the count for gamma rays was equivalent to three mSv per hour. And outside, though it was stilling raining debris, we went out and found that there was plenty of the stuff that measured around six mSv per hour."

Due to the terrific explosion, the safety of the QPB, which was supposed to be isolated from contamination, was seriously compromised.

"From then on, there was little point to our scanning at the entrance. The survey staff continued to scan the people coming in from work outside, but with a background level near the maximum detectable eighty thousand counts per second, a Geiger counter reading of seventy or eighty thousand didn't really tell you if they were contaminated or not. After that, our work on the entrance floor changed to that of simply helping them to take off their contaminated gear."

Here at the entrance was where the exhausted workers shed their protective clothing.

"All we could do was take off their helmets, then help them out of their one-piece coveralls, leaving them in their long underwear, before taking off their socks. Then we'd help the men, still dripping with sweat, out of the last layer and into new clothes before going upstairs. I'm sure many of them had radioactive contamination of varying amounts on their bodies, their faces, their hair, etc., but there was nothing we could do about it. They had work that needed doing upstairs, so they had to go upstairs! If we'd scrupulously de-contaminated them all over it would have held up the work of recovery."

At first they had supplied them with underpants, and later paper underpants, but the supply quickly ran out. After the explosion they soon had nothing at all. From then on, there was nothing for it but to carry on amid the contamination both indoors and out.

The Sergeant Major

Day 2—March 12 15:30

Sergeant Major Hidekazu Watanabe and his men of the JGSDF, who by promptly bringing their fire engines to the plant had provided what could aptly be called a lifeline, and who since then had continued to supply water to the reactors, also encountered the explosion.

"I'd just returned to the quakeproof building at the time. Five of my men had just left for Unit 1 for the next shift with some of the TEPCO people. Not long after they'd gone there was this huge bang. It was big enough to blow the walls and stairs apart.

"I'm an artillery man, and this wasn't like just *one* of the guns going off. It felt like ten of them firing at once. I was in the waiting room off to the right of the entrance and looked out of the tiny thirty-centimeter window to see white smoke and debris fly past before everything outside turned white. Inside the QPB there was stuff crashing down all over the place."

Watanabe dashed out of the room but realized he had no way to contact his men. He heard people yelling "Keep calm! Keep calm!"

"Sergeant Major, can you get in touch with your men?" asked one of the TEPCO people and there was nothing he could answer but, "No, I can't." Soon, people who'd been working outside started to flow back into the QPB.

"It blew up!" "It just exploded!" the returning workers were shouting. There were people in yellow overalls and in white Tyvek suits, some of them drenched in blood.

Are my men safe? thought Watanabe, as he promptly started to give first aid to the wounded.

"Do you have something for a splint? Find something we can use, would you? If you've got a magazine, bind it on with string. If you haven't got string, make do with a handkerchief or something." One after another, he gave instructions to the TEPCO staff around him.

"There are two layers of doors at the entrance, but nevertheless, somehow there was a sudden flood of people coming in, and it didn't look as if anyone had experience in first aid. But we soldiers get plenty of training in that, so I thought I'd better get on with dealing with the casualties right away. We had to undress them, and even cut off their gear with a craft knife. We used cardboard and string that was lying around to splint an injured leg, and all kinds of stuff like that."

But what really worried him was his own men. His frustration was so bad he hardly knew where to put himself.

Eventually, the TEPCO team got in radio contact with the TEPCO man accompanying his men, and he learned that all his own men were safe.

"I heard from the TEPCO side that their man who had gone with mine had been hit in the chest by flying debris and was injured, but the good news was that my own men were all right."

They were safe. Watanabe was relieved. Presently they appeared outside the entrance.

Watanabe hand-signaled, "Are you all right?" and his men signed back, "OK" with their fingers.

"Anyone hurt?"

At last they got indoors and, as he helped them off with their gear, he heard how close a shave it had been out there.

"They were all dripping with sweat, so I went upstairs to find something for them to drink, and then listened to their story. The explosion had been so huge that they had been unable to move, their legs were shaking so badly, they said. As for the fire engine, which had been continuously pumping water into the reactor, they said the windows had broken, the ladder and other equipment on top had been blown off, and now it was a battered mess. The passenger window had been blown in and had injured the TEPCO man sitting next to it. The JGSDF were the last to return to the QPB. All the others were back and were concerned that there was no sign of them. People were continually asking if they'd got back yet, and then, there they were! It was a relief to see them, I tell you!"

But not much later, they were told, "We're going back again. Get ready to move out," and four hours later they were back on the job of injecting water. Unsurprisingly, they were very worried.

"Sir, is it safe for us to be out here?"

"How much radiation have we been exposed to?" asked some of his men.

But Watanabe replied, "Stop fussing about whether it's bad for your health and get on with your mission."

There wasn't much else he *could* say.

Around 19:00 that night, TEPCO had a new request for Watanabe.

"Next, we're going to inject seawater into Unit 3. I'm going to lead you to a point where there is plenty of seawater, so please follow me there."

Right from the start, Watanabe had told them, "We're ready for anything. Tell us what you want us to do." He and his men were prepared to do whatever they were asked.

"Our unit from Kōriyama and the unit from Fukushima moved out on the seaward side of Unit 3 where there was a pool full of water left from the tsunami, into which we dropped a hose and sucked up the water. It was pitch dark so we couldn't see the water below, and some of the men thought we were drawing water directly from the sea. We unrolled as much hose as we could, and when we flung the intake down into the water, there was a good splash, so we were sure there was plenty of water there."

After completely submerging the ten-meter level, the tsunami had drained back into the sea but had left an enormous pool, Unit 3's nine-by-sixty meter 'reversing valve pit', full of seawater. They would use that water to cool the reactor. (See map page x.)

However, not only Unit 3 but now the water supply for Unit

2 was becoming an urgent problem. They needed to switch from cooling with the RCIC to water injection using the fire engines. They already had their hands full with Units 1 and 3 and had to decide how to allocate the limited amount of water in the reversing valve pit.

Certainly, aside from laying out a long pipeline to draw water directly from the sea, there was no other reliable source of water.

Meanwhile they had to depend on the unreliable RCIC: if it stopped, it would never start again.

Unknown to the people on the frontline, another fierce battle over the injection of seawater was being fought elsewhere. There, it was the Prime Minister's Office and TEPCO headquarters pitched against Site Superintendent Yoshida and his Emergency Response Center at the Fukushima Daiichi plant.

You can't do that!

Day 2—March 12 19:00

Immediately after having at last initiated the seawater injection in the face of such dangers as the increasing radiation since the explosion, Yoshida heard a familiar voice from the landline phone on the desk.

"Hey, there! How's the seawater injection coming along?"

The voice on the phone was that of TEPCO Fellow Ichirō Takekuro. An old hand in the narrow field of nuclear engineering, at sixty-four he was eight years Yoshida's senior, a graduate of Tokyo University's Faculty of Engineering endowed by TEPCO with the title of 'Fellow' and a vice-president's perks, and currently ensconced in the Prime Minister's Office.

Like Masao Yoshida, he was one of the few engineers in the nuclear power department of TEPCO. They were on close enough terms that there was no offense, neither intended nor perceived, in the unusually casual form of address.

Takekuro had gone straight to the point.

"It's under way," replied Yoshida calmly.

"What? Really?" replied Takekuro.

"Yes, we've already started."

The astonished Takekuro lost his presence of mind. "Who said you could do that?"

"What do you mean?"

"You can't do that. You can't."

"What's that supposed to mean?"

"You've got to stop it!"

"What are you on about? It's already running. You can't stop it now."

Yoshida was resisting this order from Takekuro. But Takekuro's next words took him quite by surprise.

"Shut up and listen, damn it! I've got the PMO on my back."

"Are you out of your mind?!"

The exchange had become extremely heated. But then the line went dead.

Yoshida constantly had to devise and apply new measures to cope with the situation with the unruly reactor. As Site Superintendent he was responsible for controlling all six reactors at the FDI plant.

Even though he could easily have been occupied in a video-conference with TEPCO HQ, or giving vital instructions to his staff at the plant, Takekuro had nevertheless taken the liberty of phoning him directly from the Prime Minister's Office. What's more, all Takekuro had wanted to convey was the miserable complaint that the PMO was getting on his back.

Why did he, the man battling on the front line, have to listen directly to the absurd requests of amateurs? Yoshida was so frustrated he wanted to scream.

Soon afterward, he was to receive a direct order from TEPCO HQ to stop the seawater injection. It was clear that the opinion of the PMO had been passed on to TEPCO HQ. But before that call came in, Yoshida laid his plans.

"We'll probably get orders from HQ to stop the seawater injection," he explained *sotto voce*. "When it comes, I will issue the order to stop so they can hear it over the video-conference link, but you don't need to respond, OK? You guys carry right on with the injection, got it?"

Even as the video-conference got underway, Yoshida carefully avoided the microphones and managed to unobtrusively explain his plans to the necessary people.

Why can't they see that a seawater injection is the only way? he thought.

"It's pretty obvious that with such a huge amount of heat to get rid of, the sea was the only way. There was a problem in that the RHR (Residual Heat Removal) system, which normally uses seawater for cooling, was also becoming unreliable. We didn't have anything like the amount of freshwater we would need, so our final conclusion was that cooling by injecting seawater was the only answer. Cooling the reactor was absolutely essential, so it was obviously the only way to go. We'd already reached that conclusion and acted on it, and then they come and tell us to stop!"

Despite the number of experts there were at TEPCO HQ who should be able to follow his reasoning, they were telling him, of all things, to stop the seawater injection. Yoshida couldn't contain his anger.

He didn't learn until much later that one of the objections from the PMO concerned their worry that injecting seawater might trigger what is called a "re-criticality" event.

After the accident, accusations of interference by the PMO were made in numerous reports on the accident. Prime Minister Kan responded to these accusations in the National Diet on May 31, 2011, at a Special Meeting of the House of Representatives' Special Committee on Reconstruction after the Great East Japan Earthquake, when responding to a question about the accident from opposition Liberal Democratic Party representative Hidenao Nakagawa.

"The problem with seawater is that, after you put it in, the water evaporates and the salt is left. There is the possibility of salt corrosion and problems like that. That's why, when you inject seawater, a careful examination of all the possible problems is the natural thing to do, isn't it? The possibility of a hydrogen explosion, or the possibility of a steam explosion, or the possibility of re-criticality, all the effects that could occur when salt gets inside . . . and I was told we had only an hour and half, so I asked all the experts there, 'Well, there you have it, work it out, will you?' At six p.m. on March 12, I personally thought that they would have to go ahead with the seawater injection, but since there were all kinds of aspects to consider, the experts should work it out properly. That was what I intended, from start to finish, and the idea that I did it all because I had some other political objective – there was absolutely nothing like that."

Despite the fact that Yoshida's decision to push ahead with the seawater injection was made at the last possible moment, it is a matter of fact that the order to stop the seawater injection was directly due to Kan's demand for more expert consultation. According to Kan himself, this expert consultation was ordered specifically because of Haruki Madaramé of the Nuclear Safety Commission.

Madaramé told me, "That's rubbish! I told him all along that a seawater injection was the only solution."

"The topic we were discussing at the time was that seawater was the only way: 'Slam it in there', I told him. I think it was Kaieda who asked about the problems of what might happen if we injected seawater, a natural question since the salt is inevitably going to pile up. If salt accumulates, it's going to hold up the flow, isn't it? So we didn't really know how long we could keep it up. I think he told the people at NISA to find out. Seawater is pretty corrosive, so we wouldn't want to keep using it for long, but at that point we couldn't afford to be choosy. Besides that, we were told to say what we liked, so I mentioned that there were some unpleasant chemical elements that can be found in seawater. Radioisotopes from artificial transmutation, I mean. They started talking about the fact that if atoms get hit by neutrons flying around, they can transform them into different isotopes, and if they were the radioactive kind, that would be nasty."

But this caused the politicians to overreact.

"It's basic nuclear physics, but as the temperature goes down, density rises, so, though it's *almost* impossible, the chance that it will go critical is not absolutely zero. Just to be sure, precautions need to be taken to prevent criticality, and as such, just to be sure, I suggested it be kept among the points to be considered. Of course, scientifically speaking, you can only say 'the probability is not zero.' But if we didn't go ahead with injecting seawater, we could have a real China Syndrome on our hands, so in my opinion, if anything was going to be top priority, it had to be cooling, and that's what I told them."

Even after the PMO's repeated meddling in the operations at the plant, there was to be more interference regarding the plan to switch from freshwater to seawater.

Madaramé continued.

"They (the Government-TEPCO Integrated Response Office)

announced that it was because I had declared there was a danger of re-criticality. So I protested. I had only said that the probability wasn't zero, but they twisted my words. To say that the probability isn't zero, and to draw attention to a danger, are two totally different things. I was speaking as a scientist, saying that mathematically the probability wasn't strictly zero. I suspect it was one of the METI bureaucrats who distorted what I said, and I still consider it an immense personal insult."

But what is most surprising is that someone as high-ranked as a prime minister should give such detailed instructions on technical matters such as the vent or the seawater injection, to the people who are supposed to be in charge (TEPCO), who have plenty of experts of their own.

Kan responded to this, thus.

"People keep complaining about 'meddling' and 'interfering' but they've got things back to front. Normally, as head of the Nuclear Emergency Response Headquarters, I would receive reports from the field on the scale of the evacuation, or the power companies would take certain measures, and I would just sit and wait, and things would be fine. According to previous legislation, the normal order of things is for the Local HQ at the Offsite Center to handle local matters and for them to come to me, the head of the NERH, to sign off on it. But in actual fact, the deputy-minister (of METI) arrived at the Offsite Center after midnight on the twelfth, only to find that the power was cut off, the people hadn't arrived, and practically speaking, the Local HQ wasn't functioning.

"Onsite, too, the law says that the normal order of things is that the power company, the people who own the operation, should run things. In this case it was TEPCO. But TEPCO couldn't even supply them with generator vehicles. Later, because they didn't have enough batteries at the plant, site chief Yoshida said they'd hooked up the batteries from their own cars, so I know the people inside the plant were working frantically. So why is it that, even on the third day, TEPCO HQ hadn't sent them enough twelve-volt batteries? Their logistics were completely incompetent."

Kan also points out that the provisions of the Nuclear Emergency Act failed to anticipate the severity of the possible emergency situations.

"These provisions were all written in response to the JCO accident (Tōkaimura 1999) and didn't take into account the conditions after an earthquake, when the staff might not be able even to assemble. So, right from the start, all sorts of thing weren't functioning properly, and we were getting desperate, so, in effect, the PM's office got on with the job. They keep on and on about 'interfering' but I wish they'd take the facts of the situation properly into account."

The PMO was forced to take matters into its own hands, whether they wanted to or not, he claimed. However, the video-conferences with TEPCO provide a video and audio record of how the PMO itself was thrown into pandemonium by the PM's 'getting desperate.'

When Fellow Takekuro returned to TEPCO HQ from the PM's office more than three hours after telling Yoshida to stop the seawater injection, he participated in a video conference and made the following statement which was recorded.

"There's a good reason they call him 'Ornery Kan'! He blows his top pretty often, and I've caught the blast six or seven times. After one of *his*, Yoshida's tempers seem almost cute, you know. Yesterday, when we were trying to decide which areas to evacuate, I was summoned, and he screamed, 'How are you gonna handle this? What are you gonna do?' And when Madaramé and I explained, he'd keep coming back with 'And what do you base that on?' or 'How do you know it'll work for sure?' The tantrums went on and on."

Ever since the earthquake, Yoshida, who had battled on without so much as a nap, hashing out plans for recovery and carrying out those plans within the plant, found that he had another battle to fight, this time against participants who actually tried to hold him back.

Last snaps

Day 2—March 12 Night

The explosion in the Unit 1 reactor building brought about some big changes at the Unit 1 and 2 control room.

On the evening of March 12, while the recovery team in the ERC was working frantically on the practical preparations for the seawater injection, Izawa finally ordered the younger operators to withdraw to the ERC. *We can't keep the youngsters here any longer,* he thought.

Now that there had been an explosion, and with radiation levels continuing to rise, they might well be faced with other unforeseen situations. About twenty of the youngest operators evacuated the Unit 1 and 2 control room.

"While they were in the control room I was responsible for them, so it was a great relief to be able to send them somewhere safer. It had been a weight on my mind all along," Izawa admitted.

Where formerly there had been nearly forty people, now there were hardly any who were not managerial level staff. As Hirano put it: "only the elderly remained." In total, there were seventeen of them.

One of the seventeen was Kazuhiro Yoshida, who had set off on the second attempt to open the AO valve for the vent. They had lost all track of time. Confined to the darkness of the control room, neither sunshine nor starry skies shone down on them. Their work consisted solely of connecting batteries to the instruments in the control room and collecting the data.

To relieve the depressing silence of the room, as dawn began to break outside, Kazuhiro tried to liven things up.

"How about taking some pictures? This could be our last chance," he called out loudly. There was no response from the exhausted men. But Izawa, Kazuhiro's senior from high school, reacted to the inauspicious words "This could be our last chance."

"No way. You'll put a jinx on us."

A digital camera for recording situations of all kinds is standard equipment in the control room. Kazuhiro ignored his senior, got out the camera and started taking snaps of each of them. As he went around, flashing away, people started waving to the camera, making thumbs-up signs and even the ubiquitous Japanese V-sign.

For these men, who had not slept since the start of the accident, with helmets and full-face masks balanced on their heads, in their blue or white Tyvek suits, or even the protective radiation suits they called their B-suits, these flash-lit scenes in the darkness of the control room might well have been the last photographs of them alive. It is hard to imagine how they felt as Kazuhiro snapped away.

"Our primary tasks were checking the pressure in the containment vessel and the water level in the reactor vessel. Every five or ten minutes we'd read them off and report them to the ERC. I started taking those pictures because we didn't know whether or not the next moment was going to be our last."

They didn't know when the next blast might come. Thus, thanks to Kazuhiro Yoshida, we have a valuable photographic record of the control room, that space where time seemed to have stood still.

On the evening of March thirteenth, Izawa and his men switched to a shift system and were able to retire in turns to the relative safety of the QPB.

Retreat

Day 3—March 13 19:00

"Except for those responsible for data collection, all personnel will retreat to the QPB. From now on we'll have rotating shifts in the control room."

According to this order from the Site Superintendent Yoshida, Izawa and his crew would now work in shifts of five men at a time. On his way from the Unit 1 and 2 control room to the QPB, Izawa saw a sight he hadn't even imagined. It was fifty-two hours, more than two days, since the earthquake.

"I hadn't been outdoors since I went into the control room on the morning before the earthquake. I'd heard about the awful shambles outside from the people coming in from the ERC, but when I saw it for myself I was astonished."

The normally neat and tidy ten-meter level was an appalling sight, strewn with the wreckage of both the tsunami and the subsequent explosion.

Even Izawa was speechless at the scale of the damage that the hydrogen blast had wrought on the upper parts of the Unit 1 reactor building. It made him think of a city battleground, devastated by an air raid.

Shocked as he was, when Izawa made his way to the QPB, he beheld a bizarre scene of a different kind. Bodies lay everywhere. This was a battlefield.

"There were slumped bodies everywhere, in the corridors, the restrooms and open spaces; anywhere room could be found. Our people and contractors lay around exhausted all over the place. It was a weird feeling. Coming back to the QPB after being in the control room, felt, to use a military metaphor, like coming back to the rear after fighting on the front line. It was a big surprise to find so many people there."

At that point there were over six hundred people in the QPB. But Izawa felt something odd about the atmosphere there. And suddenly the reason hit him.

"To use another military metaphor, I realized that most of the people there were 'non-combatants'. We had made our way back from the control room alive, only to find the place full of non-technical staff. There were loads of people just lying around, with no idea what was going on, stuffed into places out of the way, including women and contractors. We, ourselves, had escaped, if barely, with our lives, only to discover that there were all these people here that we now had to do something about."

Izawa referred to these people as "non-combatants."

"I couldn't believe how many there were. Site Superintendent Yoshida and his staff around the table in the ERC were the front line, but in the background were all these, what should I call them, 'non-combatants' taking refuge in the QPB. Well, that was a surprise, but I also began to feel that we were no longer alone there. Back in the control room we were ultimately responsible for everything, which was a very lonely feeling. But once we got back to the QPB, with Yoshida in command, there were hundreds of people on our side. In particular, the leading members of the recovery work group were working all-out to restore power despite the dangers of radiation and the threat of another hydrogen explosion. So, even though in falling back to the QPB we'd been obliged to retreat, I didn't give up hope. Back in the control room, we'd thought we were about to die, but there was no feeling like that in the QPB. *From here, we can still do it,* I thought. I remember how this strange feeling came over me that now there was hope. We still had a chance."

Forty missing!

The Colonel

Day 4—March 14 11:01

The tremendous blast came just as forty-nine-year-old Colonel Shinji Iwakuma, head of the JGSDF's Central Nuclear Biological Chemical Weapon Defense Unit went to open the passenger door of his jeep. It was one minute past eleven on the morning of March 14, and he was at the crossroads just between reactor Units 2 and 3 of the Fukushima Daiichi nuclear power plant. (See map page vii.)

There was no time even to cry out. Iwakuma couldn't tell whether he had been bounced out of his seat or whether the whole vehicle had been lifted into the air.

With the savage impact, the surroundings instantly turned grey.

Visibility was reduced to zero. Terror seemed to lurk out there in that grey world as a weird and unfamiliar noise enveloped them. It was the sound of something raining down.

Iwakuma realized it was the sound of falling debris, and that it seemed as if the debris was not simply falling, but was being deliberately directed *at* them. The rubble and fragments blown aloft by the blast continued to pour down on them. (See cover photos.)

"It lasted quite a while. I'm not sure how long, though. It may have been only seconds, or perhaps half a minute or so, but it felt as if lasted for several minutes. There were some enormous thumps too. Some wreckage hit the windshield and broke it. Then more debris fell in through the hole. There were lumps of concrete and all sorts of stuff. If we'd been hit by one of the big pieces, we'd have been done for."

Iwakuma and his men were trained soldiers. They reflexively took cover immediately.

"Keeping low and as small as possible is basic. The next thing is to try and get under cover. I got down below the passenger seat and the driver got down under his. The noise seemed unending. How much of it was the roar from the blast and how much was the noise of the rain of debris was hard to tell."

Because the blast had come from the right, Iwakuma in the passenger seat was unscathed, but the driver's side window had been blown in.

"Are you OK?" he asked the driver, as they remained under cover.

"OK, sir!" he replied. Luckily, they were both unhurt.

Who'd have thought they'd see this kind of action so soon after they arrived? Since the previous evening, March 13, Iwakuma and his team had been pumping water at another power station, the Fukushima Daini nuclear power plant eight kilometers to the south, which had been facing a similar crisis. But this morning they'd been told that there was urgent need for water supplies at the Unit 3 reactor at Fukushima Daiichi, and had just arrived there in a hurry.

"You are the only ones we can ask," the head of the Local HQ, METI vice-minister, Motohisa Ikeda had pleaded. His strained tone emphasized how serious the situation must be. But as soon as they arrived at the scene, Iwakuma and his men had been met with this tremendous explosion.

His mind was filled with conflicting thoughts on their misfortune in arriving at such a time and on their good luck in having survived.

"I was in the lead vehicle and had overtaken the water tender, so when the blast hit us I was just about to get out and guide the two trucks behind us into position. It was just as I put my hand on the door. If the door had been open, the blast would have blown it away. We were really lucky the door was still closed, I thought. The men in the tenders behind us hadn't dismounted either. If the explosion had come just a little later it would have been over for all of us."

But the damage to the truck behind was by no means minor. The roof of the cab of the nine-point-four-ton water tender was made of canvas – just a piece of fabric. The falling debris had shredded the canvas, and chunks of concrete had landed in the cab.

"There was an ordinary dump truck there, the kind used for construction, and its metal roof too was battered. It was hardly surprising that the canvas roof of the water tender had been shredded. Of course, our jeep had the same kind of canvas roof and there were lumps of concrete inside."

By the time the grey fog had dispersed, the noise had stopped too.

"Everybody out!"

"*Hai!*"

However, the blast, which had hit the driver's side, had not merely blown in the window, but had jammed the door too.

"This door looks OK. Get out this side."

Not without difficulty, he opened the passenger door and they both scrambled out. The driver's Tyvek suit was soaked in blood. He'd been hit in the back and the right thigh. It looked serious.

Smoke still wafted around. Dust and tiny metal shards still flew through the air. Though large pieces of wreckage no longer fell, the danger was not over.

Out from under the water tanker behind them crawled a soldier, favoring one leg. It seemed he had decided that was the safest place and had quickly dived for cover under the truck.

People were shouting, but it turned out that everyone was safe.

"Are you OK?"

"OK, sir," answered the limping soldier and his mates cheerfully. The men in the last truck, a second tanker, were all safe too.

The thing that worried Iwakuma most was radiation. What exactly had exploded, had radiation been released, and if so how much?

"We had to get out of there fast. All the men in the last truck had suffered bruising. One of them seemed to have injured his neck, perhaps even whiplash. They were all capable of walking out, so we evacuated on our own. By our standards, no-one was seriously hurt."

However, the counters that they carried showed that the radiation was rising extremely fast. They had to evacuate as quickly as they could.

"Fall back! Get a move on!"

"Sir!"

Iwakuma waited for the last of his men to respond, and then shouted, "Let's move!" Just at that moment, out of the corner of his eye, he spotted a figure. Through the dusty grey air he could see someone. But it wasn't just one, or even two. There were four or five. No, more. Seven or eight, at least. They appeared out of the blue, as if they had crawled out of somewhere, in their orange protective suits and masks. They were TEPCO people.

Where had they come from? Iwakuma realized he'd have to evacuate them with his own men.

"Move along there. We've got to get out of here!"

Calling to them all, with his back to the reactor building, he headed back up the road by which they had just arrived. No one spoke. Even if they'd raised their voices a little, it would have been hard to hear them through their masks. They plodded on in silence.

Behind Unit 3 they saw what looked like a fire engine.

"Let's take that and drive back!" called one of the TEPCO-suited men who'd joined them in their evacuation.

But the force of the explosion seemed to have damaged the engine and it wouldn't start, and the bodywork was severely battered from the falling debris. It couldn't be helped. They resumed walking; they must get as far from the area as possible.

"You all right? Can you keep going?"

"Keep up the pace!"

He didn't know how much they could hear through their respective masks, but he kept trying to encourage them.

"We were wearing our military ODs (Olive Drab uniform) over our Tyvek suits, with our helmets on top, so they must have known at once that we were neither reactor operators nor ordinary TEPCO personnel. The dust had pretty much settled by then."

They must have plodded seventy or eighty meters up the slope from the Unit 3 reactor when they spotted a parked dump truck.

"If the keys are in it, get that thing moving!" Iwakuma immediately ordered. Luckily the key was in the ignition.

"It works!"

This far from the explosion, the damage hadn't been so severe.

"Everybody in!"

"Get a move on!" called the soldiers to the TEPCO reactor staff, and they quickly scrambled aboard.

"Is this everyone?" Iwakuma checked.

"All accounted for," came the prompt response from the soldiers. The TEPCO people took a little longer.

"Not yet. There are more to come," they answered. Iwakuma looked back and saw they were right. About fifty meters back down the road he spotted a man slumped on the ground. And there was someone standing beside him.

"Can you back down there?" he asked the driver.

"Yes, sir," the man replied as he started to reverse the truck down the slope.

"We backed down the hill to pick the two up. Some of the men and the people from TEPCO got out, and three or four of them lifted the fellow on the ground into the truck. He was beyond walking by himself. I think he'd been hit by falling debris," Iwakuma recalls.

They couldn't take off their masks so, though he could hear the man's voice, he couldn't make out his face.

"I could hear his voice, but couldn't make out his expression. There were seven or eight of us now. We wanted to go straight back to the Offsite Center, but they wanted us to take them back to the QPB, so we detoured around there and unloaded them. The wounded were stretchered off and they all went inside. We had come here from the Offsite Center, so we had to go back there as quickly as we could to report and get treatment for our wounded. So we told them at the QPB that we were going to return to the Offsite Center, and then we set off in the truck."

Casualties

Day 4—March 14 11:01

Oh, God! We're done for! thought Site Superintendent Yoshida, as the sound and the shockwave of the explosion shook the ERC.

The pressure in the containment vessel of Unit 3 had been rising since the morning, and the danger of an explosion was increasing, so Yoshida had ordered the control room operators to withdraw to the QPB and wait it out.

The pressure had then settled down again, so he'd sent them back. And that was when the explosion occurred.

Yoshida called TEPCO HQ on the video conference link.

"HQ! HQ! We're in trouble!" he shouted. "It looks we've just had a steam explosion at Unit 3. Here at the QPB we're not sure at the moment, but it was nothing like an earthquake – there was no vertical or horizontal oscillation. I think it was the same kind as the Unit 1 explosion."

While declaring it to be of the same kind as the explosion at Unit 1, Yoshida made an unfortunate slip of the tongue and, instead of saying that it was a *hydrogen* explosion, said that it was a *steam* explosion. Just as the English word *hydrogen* is related to the Greek word *hydro* meaning water, the Japanese words for *steam* and *hydrogen* too are related. It just goes to show how unnerved he was.

"Check the parameters!"

"How's the radiation?"

The doleful silence of the ERC was suddenly replaced with a tumultuous racket.

"No change in gamma or neutron readings!"

It had been such a big explosion that Yoshida immediately thought: *I guess there'll be some dead this time.*

"Forty unaccounted for!"

As the voice thundered across the room, Yoshida froze. Hearing the figure, he thought: *Well, I guess that means I won't be getting out of here alive.*

"At that point, there were loads of people out on the site. It was me who'd sent them all out there, to go and do jobs around the site. I felt there was hardly anything left worth living for. I'd probably sent dozens of people to their deaths, so it was all *my* responsibility. I couldn't leave there alive with their deaths on my watch."

Even looking back on it at the time of interview, Yoshida was consumed with remorse.

"After the pressure went up in the Unit 3 containment vessel, I called them all back. I ordered them to take refuge here, saying it was too dangerous at the moment. But even if they came back, the seawater injection at Units 1 and 3 had to be continued. At some point we had to make arrangements for Unit 2 as well, so at some point I had to send people back out there. In fact, I'd just had a request from TEPCO HQ saying that now the pressure had settled down, wasn't it time to get back to work? Really, I'd have preferred to wait a bit longer and see how things developed, but I grudgingly sent them out with instructions to take great care. And then came the explosion. It was me that told them to go, so I thought, *They're done for! It's all my fault. . . .*"

Yoshida recalls the very words he used:

"For the time being, the pressure in the containment vessel seems to be stable, so I'd like you all to go back out and continue with the jobs you were working on."

That the explosion occurred shortly afterwards gave Yoshida pangs of conscience over his words.

The general affairs section automatically operated a system to count heads and ascertain the whereabouts of all staff whenever there was an accident or other abnormality at FDI. They would collate information from all the sections and keep a running total.

"The first thing I heard was that there were forty people missing. This only meant the number of people we had not yet *heard from*, so of course it was high at first, but still it was a huge number. I was really shocked. It sounds corny, but it gave me a kind of tight feeling in my chest, as if I couldn't breathe."

It was hardly surprising that Yoshida, on hearing the announcement from the general affairs section, should feel he'd have to 'go down with his ship'. But as time passed, the number of missing gradually dropped. As they straggled in to the QPB, some of them injured, the figure dropped to thirty, and twenty, and fifteen.

Finally the figure dropped to zero.

"I hadn't honestly expected the number to drop to zero. I was delighted. The last to be confirmed were the people from the JGSDF. They had dropped off the TEPCO staff but hadn't actually reported in at the QPB, so it took a while to confirm that they were safe. Once we knew they were safely back at the Offsite Center, we knew that no one had died. There were plenty of injuries, but the fact that there were no lives lost was a huge relief."

Operator in despair

Day 4—March 14 11:01

The Unit 1 and 2 control room had been put on a shift system the evening of the thirteenth, and when the explosion occurred, Izawa was in the ERC getting ready to relieve the previous shift.

"When the bang came, it wasn't only the shock that hit the ERC that worried me; what I saw on the TV had me worried too."

Another explosion! Are the crew in the control room safe? We must relieve them at once, thought Izawa instantly.

"With the explosion, the outdoor radiation readings shot up. At those levels we wouldn't be able to go and change shifts. When we told TEPCO HQ we were going to go, their orders were to wait, because it was too dangerous outside. I called the control room on the hotline to tell them and the operator on the other end of the line kind of choked up. . . ."

Two days earlier, Unit 1 had exploded. Now Unit 3 had blown up too. The obvious thought was that Unit 2 was next.

Even for us, being unable to relieve them was torture. I can imagine that at the other end of the hotline, when I asked them to wait a bit longer, they must have thought: *What'll become of us, then?*

The voice on the phone seemed to be choking with tears, and as if he had already made up his mind he said, "Izawa-*san*. There's no need to relieve us."

There's no need to relieve us. The words echoed in Izawa's head.

"No, no. It's just that we can't go right now," Izawa explained.

There was a moment's pause at the other end.

"It's all right. You don't have to come any more, Izawa-san."

The operator was wearing his full-face mask, which made the words "any more" seem even more indistinct. But the muffled voice struck at Izawa's heart.

"I can't forget that moment. He had made up his mind and told me he didn't need to be relieved. He was my immediate subordinate, and it's hard to live with the thought of what he went through at that moment."

What are you talking about? I'll be there in a minute! he thought and shouted "I'm the shift supervisor. The control room is *my* responsibility."

"We still hadn't got approval, but my patience had run out, and the men in the control room were going out of their minds. We didn't have time to argue about the radiation, so I just told them we were going, and a handful of us set out for the control room without permission."

Izawa and three or four of his men got into a vehicle and drove off toward the control room.

"When we got into the control room, there he was, crying embarrassedly. I didn't say anything but just thumped on his mask. Of course, he was really glad we'd come to relieve him. He was only human."

Izawa himself was only too aware, after the earthquake and tsunami, and as the situation at the plant moved from bad to worse, how encouraging it could be to know there were colleagues who would come to help.

As Izawa wordlessly thumped the operator's mask, in his mind he must have been saying: *We'd never abandon you!*

Nearing the end

On the brink

Day 4—March 14 Noon

Upstairs in the quakeproof building the atmosphere in the ERC was one of grim determination. It was already the fourth day of the accident. No one had been able to get more than a few moments of sleep and they were literally working around the clock. And now the situation was approaching its end.

When Unit 3 exploded just after 11:00 in the morning, the fire engines that they depended on for the seawater injection had been destroyed. The hoses too had been shredded and the injection of seawater, vital for cooling the reactor, had ceased. It was a dire situation.

Their inability to cool the reactor meant that the water used for cooling the hot fuel rods would evaporate, leaving them naked to the air. This meant that the fuel rods would start to react with the high-pressure steam and gradually disintegrate, bringing meltdown closer and closer.

Yoshida scheduled an examination of the reactor area for two hours later, at around 13:00, after the radiation had had time to settle. They couldn't wait any longer than that, so he made up his mind and gave instructions for the inspection of the appalling damage to the reactor building. The damage was found to be even worse than they had feared, but there was one tiny spot of good news.

The fire engine nearest the reactor building was found to be immobilized, but the two at the wharf, a short distance away on the seaward side, had escaped unharmed. These two vehicles had earlier been used to pump water from the sea, up into the reversing valve pit to keep it filled.

With these two, they could just get by.

Yoshida immediately ordered them to use the two fire engines to pump water directly from the harbor. They replaced the tattered hoses, and shortly after 15:30 the engines resumed pumping seawater.

However, the biggest problem facing them now was Unit 2. With the explosion at Unit 3, the RCIC (Reactor Core Isolation Cooling) system at Unit 2 had failed, and then the pressure in the reactor vessel had started to rise. At the same time, the water level had started to slowly drop. They tried to use the fire engines to inject seawater into the reactor but the pressure on the inside was already too high.

"The water won't go in!"

It was clear that the fuel rods were already exposed.

"The problem was that the Safety Relief Valves (SRV), which should release the excess pressure, wouldn't open, so the pressure in Unit 2 wouldn't go down. If the pressure inside the reactor went above ten kg/cm^2 the water wouldn't go in. It would stop flowing. The SRVs that should have released that pressure hadn't worked properly, time had been lost, and the pressure hadn't been released," recalled Superintendent Yoshida.

"We wanted to rig up some batteries so they could open the valves from the control room. These were valves that usually stay in the closed position all the time, so we had to force them open. But for each of them, either we couldn't connect the electric power, or else we couldn't get the compressors properly linked to get the air in; one way or another, we were stumped. There are several valves and we had a go at them one by one, but nothing seemed to work. Meanwhile the pressure in the reactor stayed high, so we could see there was no way they'd be able to inject any water."

Even unearthing a compressor from somewhere on the site and using air pressure to try and blow the valve open had met with no success. But they couldn't just give up. If they couldn't succeed in this, it meant that there was an ever-increasing likelihood that the Unit 2 containment vessel would burst.

In other words, it would be the end.

As Yoshida tells it, "It was a horrendous situation: The worst in my life. We were on the brink."

The tension in the ERC rose ever higher. When status reports on the condition of the reactor were delayed, Yoshida's reprimands flew thick and fast. "Confirmation! I need confirmation!"

There were times when people reported vaguely "I think", or "it should be, . . ." to which Yoshida would angrily retort, "I don't care what you *think*, you idiot ! What do you *know*?" or "Just because it *should be* doesn't mean it *is*, you idiot! Check it out!"

He recounted: "There were times when I was scared shitless. On the other hand, thinking about the worst that *could* happen, I guess I really would shit myself. I don't know what the others actually thought, but I reckon any real professional would know enough to be scared to death."

Yoshida had barely slept in more than three days. The reactor crews were occasionally able to lie down for a while, but it was pretty much the same as working around the clock.

"The crews working outside the reactors were amazing, you know. I was really impressed how they carried on going down there to inject water and refuel the fire engines, and the like."

The continuing crisis, which had started with the announcement of forty people unaccounted for after the explosion at Unit 3, had finally stretched Yoshida's physical condition to the breaking point.

At 18:02 a voice rang out in the ERC: "Decompression commencing!"

Ah, the pressure's dropping.

It was a memorable moment for all the staff in the ERC at the time.

It's nothing less than a miracle, thought Yoshida. And at 19:54 water injection commenced.

But there was still one thing they had to confirm. Had the safety valve opened, venting steam, thus lowering the pressure and allowing water to flow in, or was there another reason?

As Yoshida pointed out, the instruments could not be trusted.

"I immediately had the men beside the fire engine check that water was actually flowing into the reactor. I mean, it didn't matter how hard they pumped if the valve was still closed and water was not actually going in. Could they tell if water was actually flowing? I had them check the fire engine's flow gauge and feel the hoses by hand to make sure."

Water was flowing and the hoses were throbbing. Even from the outside you could tell that the water was pulsing through the hoses. That was what Yoshida had wanted them to confirm.

"I told them to look at the flow gauge and feel the flow of water in the hoses manually. After a while they reported back, first that the flow indicator was up, and then that they could also feel the flow in the hoses. You've no idea how relieved I was."

The radiation levels around the reactors were still high so they needed to keep their time there as short as possible.

"In order to limit their exposure, the workers were taking shelter behind a hut a short distance away. It was often difficult to get through, but I was able to give them instructions over a radio transceiver, and they reported back the same way."

Yoshida remembers how a wave of applause filled the ERC as the situation edged back from the brink. But fate was too cruel to let that feeling of relief last long.

Yoshida collapses

Day 4—March 14 21:35

When the radiation meter at the main entrance to the Fukushima Daiichi site, nine hundred meters from the reactors, reached five hundred microSieverts per hour (μSv/h) the time was about 21:35.

The pressure in the Unit 2 containment vessel, which had begun to fall, started rising again. It was as if the capricious reactor were toying with these mere mortals.

At 22:50, TEPCO HQ announced to a press gathering that, since the pressure in the Unit 2 containment vessel had risen abnormally, they had submitted drafts of notification to the Prime Minister in accordance with Article 15 of the Nuclear Emergency Act. In spite of the determined efforts of the reactor staff, the pressure was not falling, and the crisis continued.

The executives already sitting at their conference table were exhausted. At 23:46 the pressure in the containment value had reached seven hundred and fifty kilopascals (kPa, approx. seven point five atmospheres), almost twice its designed operating pressure, so it would hardly be surprising if something unusual occurred.

On the other hand, at Unit 2, a vent had been successfully carried out the previous day. The radiation levels at this reactor were nowhere near as high as those at Unit 1, so the electric MO valve had been opened manually, and the pneumatic AO valve briefly opened with an external air injection. However, because of an electrical fault, believed to have been caused by the blast at Unit 3, the AO valve closed again and, despite the desperate efforts of the recovery team, it never re-opened.

Conditions deteriorated seesaw style, one step forward, one step back. The senior staff, though none of them dared to mouth the words, were well aware that they might well be on a slippery slope to catastrophe. In view of the danger that the containment vessel might rupture, Yoshida decided to send the contractor staff offsite.

He went out of the ERC into the corridor and announced in a loud voice, "I want everyone who is not directly involved in current operations to leave temporarily. Thank you for all your efforts so far. I am deeply grateful."

In the corridor there were people lying everywhere, still in their Tyvek suits and sleeping like logs. Some slept with their heads on their knees, others slumped against walls or squeezed into tiny corners. It looked like a field hospital.

They were jolted awake by Yoshida's voice and started to listen. Every one of them had already sensed that things were coming to a conclusion. But going home meant leaving the safety of the QPB for the danger of the contaminated outdoors. Then again, it was a risk they had to take in order to evacuate the site.

"Thank you very much, all of you!"

The sight of Yoshida bowing deeply to them all confirmed to the contractors' employees, who had worn themselves out trying to restore the plant, that the end was near.

When he returned to his desk a while later, in the pre-dawn hours, several people noticed that Yoshida wasn't quite himself. His face lad lost all its vigor and his expression seemed vacant. This was quite unlike him.

Without warning, he pushed his chair back and rose groggily to his feet. One hundred and eighty four centimeters tall and weighing eighty three kilograms, the well-built Yoshida rose from his seat like a ghost, immediately turned his back to his desk and slumped down, cross-legged on the floor.

His head drooped slowly forward. With his eyes closed, he remained motionless. His arms were wrapped around his long crossed legs. It looked almost as if he were doing Zen meditation.

So, this is it . . . It's all over. . . .

All those around him knew that's what this meant. No one said a word. They watched Yoshida in silence. It was enough to impress everyone in the ERC with the gravity of the situation.

Yoshida's body language spoke eloquently of the coming of the end.

One of the first to notice Yoshida's transformation was fifty-one-year-old Noriko Igari, whose desk stood behind his, in the Corporate Communications Department.

"At that moment, I thought immediately that the end must be near. Mr Yoshida, who had been sitting at his desk for some time, suddenly stood up, only to slump down below the edge of his desk, cross-legged on the floor. For quite a while he just sat there, with his head bowed and his eyes closed. My first thought was *Ah, the plant is done for.*"

Igari was neither a technician nor a nuclear specialist. Though she could guess at the situation in the plant, she hadn't been informed of the details. For three . . . five . . . ten minutes, nothing changed. Igari watched him silently. Her desk in the Corporate Communications Department was barely five meters from his. Ever since the earthquake, no matter how exhausted he was, Yoshida had never shown any sign of his tiredness, until this moment when he finally reached his limit.

All this time, while Yoshida's head was bowed he had been thinking about just one thing.

"I'd been running through the people who I could count on to stand by me right to the very end," he recalls.

"By this time I was sure the plant was completely doomed. I couldn't even sit in my own chair any longer. I pushed it out of the way and sat on the floor. No, it wasn't your proper lotus position; I just crossed my legs and leaned back against the desk. There was nothing more I could do. The rest was up to Buddha and the gods."

Yoshida had reached his limit. He recalled his thoughts during that time.

"I considered how many people I'd need to man the plant, and what they'd have to do. I went through them in my mind, one by one. Since I'd joined TEPCO, I'd spent quite a lot of time at Fukushima Daiichi. I'd been posted there repeatedly since I was young, and it all added up to more than ten years in total, so there were lots of people there that I'd worked with over the years."

And one by one, he brought them to mind, he said.

"I was wondering how to get the men at the plant to stand by me at the end and whether I'd even need to ask. It all depended on how things worked out for the plant itself.

"I had to think about how many men I'd need to continue with the water injection, and which of them I could ask. There were all sorts of things to be done. In the final contingency, I'd have to stay here myself, whatever happened to the plant, I thought. I went through all the people who would stick with me to the end, and even die there. The generator team was no longer as important as the recovery team who were injecting the water, or the fire-fighting team with their pumps. Once we'd got this far, theirs was the major part of the task. I'd worked in the repairs section at FDI in my early thirties, so there were loads of people I'd worked with there, and who came to mind."

The first that he recalled was the leader of the recovery team, who happened to be the same age.

"There were two leaders in the recovery team, actually, and he was one of them. We were just the same age so we'd done all sorts of things together. He was the first that came to mind and I knew he'd face death with me."

As Yoshida spoke of this one who would be willing to die with him and that one who would stay with him to the end, and how he had recalled them, words for death and dying came repeatedly.

"It was mostly people of my own age that came to mind, those who had shared my early years in the company. As they filed through my mind, while on one hand I felt sorry for dragging them down with me, on the other hand it couldn't be helped. We couldn't just stop injecting water. We had to go on. The whole time I was thinking how eventually there'd be nothing I could do but ask them to sacrifice their lives.

Yoshida has no recollection of how long he sat there and pondered.

"I don't know how long I sat and thought. I can't even guess. I simply have no memory of time. But then, since there was nothing

I could do, I made up my mind to just sit and wait for the data. That's all there was to be done – wait for things to get better. If we didn't get any report of improvement, we just had to resign ourselves and carry on with the recovery operations as long as we survived."

Once he was resolved to face death himself, it's perhaps natural that the old friends who had shared Yoshida's work over his long career in the company should spring to mind.

Ms. Igari recalled what happened next.

"After that, Mr Yoshida collapsed onto his side. I was alarmed. Even he had a limit, I thought. He lay like that for some time. We were all depending on him. He was an unpretentious man, honest and direct. He was physically a big man, but as a person too he was somehow larger than life. Whatever happened, he never evaded the issue, so everyone trusted him completely. And now, here he was, like this. I thought the end had come. After a while, one of the other people from my department went over to him as he lay by his desk, tried to encourage him and asked if he could manage. It must have lasted about half an hour."

This man who had fought to protect the nation of Japan was on his last legs.

The Prime Minister's Office

Frenzy in Tokyo

Day 4—March 14 **Almost midnight**

When Haruki Madaramé, head of the Nuclear Safety Commission, received the news that Unit 2 had at last started to stabilize, March 14 was coming to a close, and he decided to get some rest. He had been up since the start of the disaster and the sleepless nights were taking their toll. He had been getting unsteady on his feet and had been advised by those around him to take a rest, and so he spent a couple of hours lying on a sofa in a room used by his deputy as NSC chief, Yutaka Kikuta.

But at around 02:00 in the morning Madaramé was abruptly woken. He was informed that the pressure at Unit 2 had started to rise again, the situation was looking more serious, and that he was summoned to see the Prime Minister in his reception room.

The PM wasn't there when Madaramé entered the room. Instead there was a gaggle of government officers: Chief Cabinet Secretary, Edano; Deputy Chief Cabinet Secretary, Fukuyama; Minister Kaieda from METI; Special Advisors to the Prime Minister, Hosono and Terata; as well as the politicians, Masaya Yasui, chief of METI's Energy Conservation and Renewable Energy Department at the Agency for Natural Resources and Energy; and Tetsurō Itō, Deputy Chief Cabinet Secretary for Crisis Management. Edano and Kaieda immediately asked Madaramé for his opinion.

"TEPCO say they want to evacuate everyone from FDI. What do you think?"

Edano and Kaieda looked grim. On hearing the question put like that, Madaramé couldn't believe his ears.

Only minutes earlier, the two ministers, Edano and Kaieda, had received a phone call from Masataka Shimizu, TEPCO president and CEO, informing them that conditions at Unit 2 were very serious and that TEPCO were considering evacuating the plant if the situation continued to deteriorate. Shimizu had made his announcement and sought the ministers' approval. He had not made any mention of leaving a minimal maintenance crew, so the ministers had assumed his announcement to mean a complete evacuation, and consequently had immediately summoned Madaramé for his opinion.

Madaramé was astounded. A complete evacuation was unthinkable. It would mean abandoning control of the reactors and allowing the whole plant to run wild.

Such a thing was unforgiveable. If TEPCO actually went ahead and abandoned the plant it would mean they were completely deserting their duty as operators of the whole enterprise; simply throwing in their hand. That was as bad as betraying the whole country. Madaramé wasn't merely astounded, he was furious.

Yasui joined him in expressing his opinion.

"Once the plant is abandoned it will be impossible to get near the reactors again."

"After TEPCO abandons the plant, you can't expect the JSDF or the US military to come in and clear it all up. That's out of the question. The company must take care of the plant right to the very end."

"The QPB has filters and air-recycling for complete protection against radioactivity so they should be able to last there for a while yet," they insisted.

The QPB still held around six hundred people, and Site Superintendent Yoshida was already planning to have all but a skeleton maintenance crew moved to the Fukushima Daini plant less than ten km away, but Madaramé and Yasui (in Tokyo) knew nothing of that.

The people in the PM's reception room were unanimous that a complete evacuation was unthinkable.

At 03:00, Kan, who had been sleeping on a sofa in the reception room in the rear of his office, was woken by one of his secretaries. Kaieda had an urgent message for him.

"TEPCO say they would like to evacuate the plant. How would you like us to handle it?"

TEPCO, evacuate? Kan was horrified at the sudden news. If they abandoned the plant what would happen to Japan?

Kan, who since the beginning had been unable to keep that ultimate disaster scenario out of his mind, later recalled this stage of the crisis.

"Ever since the accident began, I'd been thinking about the worst possible case. A thermal power station or an industrial complex can become a disaster if the fuel tanks catch fire, but at some point the fuel will burn out. That's where a nuclear power station is completely different. You can run away when the danger reaches a certain level, but a nuclear plant will not burn out. And without anyone there to control the reactors, once one of them gets knocked out, in due course they will all be knocked out. That means the total of ten reactors at Fukushima Daiichi and Daini plants plus their eleven pools of spent fuel rods would all be done for. Those were the basic figures I had in mind."

The Prime Minister spelled out more of that ultimate scenario he imagined.

"First of all, never in the world has a containment vessel exploded. That's partly because Chernobyl didn't even *have* a containment vessel. But in terms of quantities, I was aware that it would be on a scale well beyond that of Chernobyl.

"Chernobyl didn't go wrong because the cooling failed but because the nuclear reaction got out of control and went bang. And Chernobyl was a graphite-moderated reactor, so once the graphite started burning it all went up at once. Our problem was that the amount of nuclear material in the Fukushima Daiichi and Daini plants' ten reactors and eleven pools of spent fuel rods totaled at least ten times as much as in Reactor Four, the one which blew up, at Chernobyl. What would happen if all of that got out of control? What would happen to Japan then? That's what had been on my mind all along."

Kan also tells of the loneliness of being the leader of a nation.

"The prime minister's residential quarters are just next door but I didn't get back there for a whole week, and spent the nights in my overalls under a blanket on a sofa in the reception room beyond my office. Whenever I was alone, this kind of thing was always on my mind. What would become of Japan? I honestly felt shivers down my spine. At Chernobyl, they sent in the military with loads of cement and heaped it up into a sarcophagus. And a lot of people died from doing that. They dealt with it by throwing their military at it and taking heavy casualties. Even I'd heard all about it, so I couldn't stop thinking about how things would go if TEPCO decided to do a bunk."

Needless to say, if it came to that, the capital, Tokyo, would be doomed too.

"It's obvious. There's nothing scarier than a nuclear reactor out of control. There's no such thing as martial law in Japan, so there was no knowing how long it would take to evacuate the local people, or what scale the evacuation would have to take. Up to then even I'd had to be very careful what I said. For example, just as it was a personal problem for everybody, if things came to a head, then there was the Emperor and the Imperial family to think of, too.

"After the problem of evacuating the plant came up on March 15, I addressed the ministers and cabinet advisors on the subject for the first time. I told them that abandoning the plant was unthinkable, and asked them if they realized what would happen if the plant were abandoned. Until that point it was the elephant in the room, and I'd refrained from broaching the subject," he recalled, looking back on the excruciating dilemma he had faced.

"Shunsuké Kondō, the head of the cabinet's Atomic Energy Commission, estimated that the radius of the evacuation area would need to be about two hundred and fifty kilometers. That would include the whole of the Kantō plain (i.e. extended Tokyo area), all the northeastern Tōhoku region except for Aomori (at the northern tip of the main island of Honshū), and even parts of Niigata in the west (on the Japan Sea coast). Just think what that would mean! Two hundred and fifty km would mean about fifty million people. That's forty percent of the nation! That's what would happen if they just walked off and left the plant to itself. I knew we had to do everything we could to stop them. We had no choice but to literally risk our own lives, and that included me, I thought."

It was about an hour later, a little after 04:00 that TEPCO chairman, Mr Shimizu, was summoned to the PM's Office.

Gathered in the Prime Minister's reception room were the PM

and his Chief Cabinet Secretary, Edano; METI Minister, Kaieda; the PM's Special Advisor, Hosono; Deputy Chief Cabinet Secretary, Fukuyama; and Madaramé.

The politicians sat along one side of the long main table while the technical experts including Madaramé and the ministers sat facing them. Prime Minister Kan took the seat at the head of the table where he could overlook both sides.

TEPCO headquarters are in Uchisaiwaichō, Chiyoda ward, only a kilometer and a half from the PM's Office. By car, it would take less than ten minutes. Shimizu arrived not long after everyone else was seated at the main table. Kan went straight to the point.

"Is TEPCO is going to evacuate the FDI plant?" he asked.

Shimizu's reply took everyone by surprise.

"We have no intention of evacuating the plant."

What? They're not going to evacuate, after all? After all of us turned out to an emergency meeting in the middle of the night? All those at the meeting must have thought very much the same thing.

"When Shimizu told us they had no intention of evacuating the plant, I felt kind of deflated. It was just what I'd thought in the first place," Madaramé recalls. Up to that point, I'd been telling the politicians that TEPCO were going to evacuate all their staff from the plant. I didn't actually know what the radiation levels were at the plant. Nor did I know how long the air-filters at the QPB would last. But I hadn't heard of any further incidents, so I'd suspected it was just TEPCO weeping and wailing about how there was nothing they could do. I had intended to ask Shimizu why they had to evacuate. As far as I could see, it was a crazy idea. So when he walked in and told us they had no intention of evacuating the plant, it was a huge surprise. It was quite a let-down, in fact. All along I'd had a suspicion it was nonsense. I mean, they couldn't just abandon the plant – it was ridiculous!"

Madaramé listened to the rest of what Shimizu had to say.

"He spoke in a small voice, almost whispering, and announced that they had no intention of evacuating the plant. I'd been unable to believe that they'd really abandon the plant, and the politicians had kept asking me if we could allow them to go ahead. The way they had continually asked me the same question, I myself had come to believe that they were going to completely evacuate the site. I hadn't had any direct phone call myself, but since a number of politicians told me they had heard it directly from TEPCO, I was taken in.

"I must say, TEPCO definitely sent these politicians a misleading message with their phone calls."

The combination of Shimizu's lack of explanation and the misunderstanding among the politicians who *were* informed, later led to the controversy over the 'complete evacuation', which was discussed even in the Diet. Madaramé blamed TEPCO for the confusion.

"Let me make it clear," he explained. "I very much sympathize with the politicians. They can't be expected to understand the technical side. And I was confined to the Prime Minister's office the whole time, so I was wrapped up in the same state of mind as the people there. They had an extremely deep distrust of both TEPCO and NISA (the Nuclear Industrial Safety Agency). The PMO didn't trust TEPCO in the least and I can well understand why they regarded everything coming out of TEPCO with suspicion."

At this meeting in the PM's office, Kan announced to Shimizu: "You are failing to communicate adequately. In order to handle the situation appropriately, TEPCO and the government will combine forces and set up a joint-command at the TEPCO headquarters."

This was not a request but a notification, and there is no doubt that it was a result of the PMO's distrust of TEPCO.

Histrionics

Day 5—March 15 05:30

Prime Minister Kan appeared in TEPCO's Emergency Response room on the second floor of the TEPCO headquarters in Tokyo about an hour later, shortly after 05:30, having arrived by car. After working around the clock for days, everyone was totally exhausted.

Kan accepted the microphone from the chairman of the meeting, Special Advisor Hosono. "The press have all gone now, haven't they?" he checked, before launching into his now-famous, ten-minute speech.

"I'm sure you all know what the current situation at FDI means," he began.

"Until now the government has had its own Nuclear Emergency Response Headquarters, as specified by law, but it's clear that it would be advisable to form a Government-TEPCO Integrated Response Office in co-operation with the operating company. Under the law, I, Prime Minister Kan, am entitled to issue direct commands to the operating company. I will head this office myself."

The speech was broadcast by video-conference not only to Yoshida's emergency response center at FDI but simultaneously to FDN (the Fukushima Daini plant), to the Local HQ at the Offsite Center in Ōkuma, and to the TEPCO nuclear plant at Kashiwazaki-Kariwa. Quite a few people were already hastily scribbling notes as the PM spoke.

"The deputy heads will be Minister Kaieda and Mr Shimizu of TEPCO."

Kaieda leapt to his feet and bowed deferentially. Kan's tone grew steadily more intense.

"The damage resulting from this accident is enormous. If things go on like this, Japan is done for. Abandoning the plant is unthinkable! You must risk your lives on it if necessary."

At the other end of the video-conference link, Kan was visible only from behind, but his voice resounded through the mike. With his left hand on his hip, he turned and addressed people around the room as he lectured on.

Needless to say, though Yoshida and his team, battling on the frontlines at FDI, could not see the expression on Kan's face, they could hear his rising fury and his next words struck them to the quick.

"If you abandon the plant, TEPCO will be destroyed. You can run, but you'll never get away!"

Run? Who's he talking about? Who does he say is running away? Kan's words changed the atmosphere in the ERC at FDI.

What's that idiot driveling on about?

Like Yoshida, all the people who'd been struggling to handle the situation at the plant, continually on a knife-edge between life and death, had already determined to stay to the end. And now their own prime minister was telling them "You can run, but you'll never get away!"

"I myself visited the plant and discussed the situation with the Site Superintendent. But the information I get from you is always too late. TEPCO's data is inaccurate, and even wrong. Even though the hydrogen explosion at Unit 1 was broadcast on TV, your report didn't reach the government until an hour later. Don't just deal with what's already on your plate: get your act together, forecast the possibilities and deal with them now!"

Perhaps it was his agitation, but his language was getting wilder.

"All those managers nearing sixty can go to the site and die on the job. I'll go myself. All you top executives, too. Say your goodbyes!"

There was a stir among those listening to the speech over the video-link. It was conduct unheard of for a prime minister.

"If you abandon the plant, TEPCO will be destroyed," Kan repeated, and after looking around at the assembled management staff, continued, "Why are there so many of you here anyway? You only need half a dozen to decide the important stuff. Stop screwing around and get me a smaller room!" Now he was absolutely furious.

The personnel in the Emergency Response room at TEPCO HQ were dumbstruck at the PM's rage, but those who heard the irate yells thunder around the ERC at FDI were thrown into a strange atmosphere of anger and futility.

That was when Yoshida, who had been sitting at the conference table in the middle of the ERC, turned his back to the screens and cameras of the videoconference and stood up.

What's he up to?

The people around him watched as he lowered his trousers, exposing his underpants, and proceeded to adjust his shirttails. Even turning your back to a superior is taboo in Japan, but Yoshida had shown the Prime Minister his butt!

Damn idiot, shooting his mouth off! What does he know? is probably a close approximation to what Yoshida would like to have said. For Yoshida, risking his life on the site, his PM, his senior at Titech (who in normal circumstances should command respect) made him feel both desolated and angry.

The prime minister later explained what he had really meant.

"That's not quite what I meant when I said *You'll never get away!* It wasn't the personal *you,* but the more general *you*: The whole nation of Japan. Japan was faced with destruction, so what

I meant was that the nation as a whole couldn't escape unharmed. As far as I was concerned, that included me. I wouldn't have been able to escape either.

"I wasn't referring directly to the people on site in Fukushima but simply speaking as prime minister of the nation. What I wanted to say then was that Japan couldn't just throw in its hand and give up on getting the situation under control. We couldn't leave it for some other country to save the day. It was the nation of Japan that couldn't escape from the problem. I wasn't trying to blame anyone."

That's how Kan remembers the comments that so appalled the people on the ground when they heard them over the video-link.

Last Goodbyes

Evacuate!

Day 5—March 15 06:30

Ikuo Izawa frequently remembers the scene.

"Unit 2 suppression chamber showing zero pressure!"

His voice rang across the ERC. The rest of the staff didn't so much reply as simply gulp. It was a little after 06:30 on the morning of March 15. Moments before, the ERC had been engulfed in the noise of another blast. Obviously something had exploded.

Where is it this time?

As the ERC tensed, Site Superintendent Yoshida shouted, "Check the parameters!"

"*Hai!*" came the response.

Izawa, at the shift supervisor's desk, immediately called the control room. Since the evening of the thirteenth, two days before, they had been switching shifts every few hours in the Unit 1 and 2 control room.

At that moment there were four operators there under the leadership of Hirano. By the light of their flashlights in the blackout that had followed the explosion, they were connecting the batteries to the instruments, one by one, to read off the parameters. That was when they discovered that the pressure in the suppression chamber read zero.

"Unit 2 suppression chamber pressure reads zero!"

Hirano had immediately called Izawa. Still grasping the receiver, Izawa relayed the information to the ERC in a voice that boomed to the very corners of the room. With Units 1 and 3 having suffered hydrogen explosions, they had all been thinking that Unit 2 might be next.

That time had come. The whole of the power generation team thought it was all over. The suppression chamber is a huge steel torus in a room directly below the containment vessel. It is half full of water and is used to condense steam exhausted from the containment vessel upstairs. (See diagram page ix.)

Steam that has leaked from the reactor core is released underwater in this suppression chamber to cool and condense. As long as the torus didn't leak, a highly radioactive release could be avoided. However the news that the pressure inside the torus was now zero meant that the suppression chamber, which had been their last hope, might have a hole in it.

Later inspections revealed that at Unit 2, where the attempts to vent had failed, the explosion had caused some additional damage, and more radioactivity had been released than at any of the other reactors.

This could be the situation we've been afraid of, thought Izawa, still clutching the phone as he stared out across the suddenly hectic ERC.

He lost track of time until Yoshida's bellow brought him around, roaring instructions.

"All work groups! Pick skeleton crews and evacuate everyone else!"

Yoshida had finally ordered his work groups to evacuate the plant and leave the smallest possible teams behind.

The people in the ERC had just been subjected to Kan's harangue. Only half an hour had passed since they had been knocked into a stupor by the PM's diatribe. The very people who were already risking their lives had apparently been told to go and die on the job.

Their stupefaction had not yet dissipated and the atmosphere was fraught, but now the worst-case scenario was upon them.

"Group leaders, appoint essential staff," added Yoshida. Now that Yoshida had finally ordered an evacuation, Izawa suddenly had a most unusual feeling. It occurred to him that, in a certain sense, Yoshida was actually relieved.

"At this point, there were still more than six hundred people in the QPB, including many who were not even technical staff. I'm sure Yoshida wanted the non-technical staff evacuated as soon as possible. The problem was that the level of contamination outside the building was still rising, so he couldn't send them out there either. But at this point the situation changed and it became a matter of the lesser of two evils, so Yoshida ordered us all to fall back to the Fukushima Daini plant, leaving minimal crews to keep things running. The reason I'd thought that Yoshida was, in a certain sense, actually relieved to have ordered the evacuation was that I'd been in much the same the situation myself when I had been bottled up with my colleagues as shift supervisor in command of the control room."

Izawa appreciated the heartache of being responsible for the life and death of his men, and empathized with Yoshida.

In fact, he himself was strangely pleased with the fact that Yoshida had been able to issue the orders for an evacuation. This empathy must have sprung from his own experience, living on the edge in the control room, ever since the earthquake.

The Safety Officer

Day 5—March 15 07:00

"Pick skeleton crews and evacuate everyone else!" The command had stirred the QPB into a kind of frenzy. There were, needless to say, no standard specifications on what constituted a minimal crew. The line between what was essential and what they could manage without was vague. In most cases, the people in the frenetic QPB had to make up their own minds.

Izawa decided that he wanted everybody without technical skills to leave the building. He spoke to a young man in front of him.

"Hey, you! What are you doing? Get out of here!"

"No, sir. I'm staying."

"Don't be stupid! You're young. Get out!"

"No, sir! I'm staying!"

"It's an order. Get out, now!"

In a similar manner, Izawa managed to dismiss the members of the generator team, one by one.

"Thank you for everything."

"I'm sorry I couldn't do more."

The youngsters excused themselves politely and left, some with tears in their eyes.

But it wasn't only the younger staff that evacuated. There were veterans whom Izawa had been sure would stay, who had packed their bags and gone.

Under any circumstances, the brink of death is cruel. Kazuhiro Yoshida, who had risked his life on the second attempt at a vent, was in the ERC with Izawa at this point. He recalls how he tried to avoid seeing who left and who stayed.

"When everyone started to move out, there was a huge commotion. Loads of people were leaving, and wouldn't be around anymore. I was one of those who told the younger people to get out. There were some younger ones who said they'd stay, but I was sure they were only saying so out of a sense of duty, and in their hearts they really wanted to go. Of course they did. They were young. And when we gave them direct orders to leave, they left."

That scene on the brink of death is one that Yoshida says he prefers not to recall.

"I didn't want to think about who had left and who had remained, because I didn't want any bad feeling about it later. Some of the people who I'd long seen as technicians to the core, who I trusted, had just disappeared, so I decided not to dwell on it.

"Quite a few of the older staff evacuated too. Personally I'd thought that those with technical skills should stay. But most of them took themselves off to FDN. Well, I guess we're all only human," he reflected with feeling.

It must have been a terrible experience, testing the limits of his humanity. Everyone has their own family, their own life to live. Even though they may work together in the same workplace, they all have their own circumstances and their own burdens to bear.

That all these different people were affected by a multitude of different circumstances and made different decisions on evacuating to FDN merely showed that they were human.

At the same time, there was one person moving against the flood of people. The woman trying to get upstairs to the ERC was forty-nine-year-old Mari Satō of the Disaster Prevention and Safety Group.

As its name suggests, the group was responsible for the safety and orderly movement of employees in case of a disaster. It was she who, even when the building was still shaking from the earthquake, had leapt to the emergency announcement system and had broadcast the command to evacuate the building to everyone there.

However, panels had begun to crash down from the ceiling, ripping out the wiring and abruptly ending her broadcast after that single command. Since then she had remained in the QPB, helping with various tasks including looking after the outdoor workers, supplying meals, and even re-fuelling the fire engines running at the reactors. And she was by no means the only woman left in the QPB.

"Everyone was filthy and in a terrible mess. Nobody could take a bath – there wasn't any water for that. And because the ceilings and all had fallen down, everyone had their heads covered in dust and couldn't do anything about it. The men were unshaven and couldn't even wash their faces; the women had straggly hair hanging down, and were without a trace of make-up. If anyone got hold of a medical mask they'd wear it just to hide their face. Then the toilets wouldn't flush, and everyone had to sleep on the floor, all together, higgledy-piggledy. It was awful," she explained.

Then, on March 15 came Site Superintendent Yoshida's order to evacuate. Satō had been down on the first floor, so she hadn't heard the announcement directly, but as people started to flood down the stairs she realized what was happening.

The equipment for going outdoors was all assembled on the first floor. People lined up to put on Tyvek suits, full-face masks and then plastic covers for their footwear.

But if everyone leaving the site wore a mask, there wouldn't be any left for the people who remained to work on the plant. No one would be able to get near the reactors anymore.

Some of the masks were hidden away to be used by the people who would stay behind. There were not enough left for everyone, so there was a bit of a scramble for them.

Those who were unable to get a mask covered their mouths with handkerchiefs for the dash to the bus or to shared rides in the employees' own cars.

As she watched the exodus, Satō remembered that there were some younger people in her own section who were still upstairs in the ERC. It wouldn't do to have them risk their young lives with the old folks, she thought as she dashed up the stairs. When she entered the room, she found Yoshida and the senior staff sat around the conference table, in silence.

"Honestly, Yoshida and about fifty of the managerial staff were just sitting there without a word to say. It wasn't just quiet; it was silent! Until then there had always been a restless bustle in the ERC, so the difference was striking."

From the entrance she could see, on the far side of the conference table under the video conference screen on the farthest wall, a group of three junior staff sitting in a circle on the floor. They were from the fire-fighting squad.

Satō circled the table and approached them under the screen.

"The others are all downstairs dressed and waiting to go," she chivvied them, but there was no response. "The rest of the fire-fighting squad are ready. You must go and join them. They are on the bus already," she continued, but none of them moved. They didn't even bother to reply.

"I really thought that all of us who stayed behind were going to die there, so I didn't want the younger ones dying there with us. The senior staff had their own responsibilities so they had no choice, but knowing those kids were just going to die there without a fight, I couldn't bear to see them stay behind. All the others had split up and gone downstairs, and left the QPB, so I tried to persuade them to hurry up because the others were waiting, but they wouldn't move."

They had resolved to stay, she thought, and she realized the strength of their commitment.

"I was convinced that the plant was doomed, but that they would be able to come back to restore it someday. I was brought up in an age when everybody read *Kike Wadatsumi no Koe* (a famous postwar compilation of letters and notes written by college students sent to their deaths in World War II) so I was well aware of the tragedy of young people throwing their lives away in suicide attacks. So there was no way I was going to let *these* youngsters waste their lives."

She screamed at them in a voice that surprised even Satō herself.

"There'll be work for you later, when they come back to clear up!"

Her voice was loud enough to echo throughout the ERC. She was desperate. If she didn't tell them, they'd continue to refuse to evacuate, and there was no time to be lost.

You need to devote your lives to the recovery, was what the older Satō wanted them to understand. Just as if those young soldiers in the Pacific War could instead have been used to rebuild the nation.

However, Satō's voice also reached the ears of the senior staff around the conference table. For them, the words "clear up" implied no less than their own demise.

"I think the senior staff at the conference table had all already accepted that they were going to die on the job, and, in fact, I agreed that they had to stay right to the end. I felt sorry for them, but I was convinced that the younger people had to be sent home to fight another day. The older men were going to die anyway; that couldn't be helped. Seeing them all there with the same thought in mind, it looked as if they were all, figuratively, dressing for a ritual mass suicide," she recalled.

The three finally rose to their feet. Satō had at last spurred them into action. As she led them to the exit she exchanged a few words with the head of her Disaster Prevention and Safety Group, words which to this very day she regrets.

"I unthinkingly suggested that he come with us. Even now, I can't think what made me say something so stupid to someone who'd already made up his mind to stay.

"He didn't know what to say and just mumbled something. When all the other section heads were staying behind, he couldn't be the only one to evacuate, but I had to open my big mouth and put my foot in it!"

Site Superintendent Yoshida had been watching all of this. His expression was completely tranquil, she said.

"Mr Yoshida had been watching us calmly. I'm sure he was already completely resigned. He always sat up straight. He wasn't the kind to fidget. He just sat there and watched us unperturbed. I knew it was the last I'd ever see any of them again, so I turned to face them, not just him, bowed a farewell to them all and left the ERC."

After her deep bow, Satō never looked back.

"I turned away. There was an air of sanctity there. The fifty-odd men around the table seemed like samurai about to perform ritual suicide, facing death serenely. It would have been discourteous to turn and gawk. The proper thing for a common soldier like me to do was to hurry away. It was so quiet in there. . . ."

Everyone but the technicians required for the restoration of the plant had been evacuated.

Mari Satō never expected to see any of them again.

The Fifty

Day 5—March 15 Morning

The ERC was silent. After the earlier pandemonium, the tranquility was unbelievable. Strangely there was no feeling of desperation.

Izawa recalled thinking that the people he needed to stay had stayed.

"After I'd finished seeing everyone off, I looked around and found that plenty of people from the power generation team were still there. *Wow! So many?* I thought. Of course the technicians in the generation team were the people we most needed to stay and help, but nevertheless I was pleased to see there were so many. There must have been a couple of dozen. It was a nice surprise."

The quiet in the ERC at that time is something that Izawa will never forget.

"I mean, there was this huge whoosh as everyone evacuated the building, and then it all stopped. After that, once it was over and only the essential people were left, it was really hushed. All the people who'd stayed kind of looked around at each other without saying anything. It wasn't a feeling of desperation, you know. It'd be weird to say they were smiling, but there was a special kind of mood in the room."

Site Superintendent Yoshida broke the silence and addressed them abruptly. "How about something to eat?"

Considering the severity of the situation, his words seemed so out of place, but the strained atmosphere of being continually one misstep from death was gone in a flash. This was exactly the kind of thing that made Yoshida different from other people.

At his command, people started to rummage around for things to eat.

"I wonder if there's anything to eat in here."

"Yes, look what I've found!"

"Here you are. Have one of these!"

Biscuits and crackers appeared from nooks and crannies, and were passed out to everyone.

"When Yoshida said 'How about something to eat,' I realized I'd done exactly the same thing myself," recounted Izawa with a laugh. "I'd said the same thing when everything had gone really quiet while we were holed up in the control room. It was a way to change the atmosphere, a way to break the ice, I guess. When Yoshida said it, a kind of roar broke out and everyone got up and started rummaging around in drawers looking for food. Not that there was anything but emergency rations, and for drinks there was only bottled water."

While poking around, someone even found some iodine tablets.

"Hey, want some of these?" he called out, and the pills were shared out with the food.

"'Sure! I could eat anything,' they'd answer. It was somehow refreshing. We'd realized we were all committed now. The silence had dragged on; nobody felt like chatting with HQ in Tokyo, and it felt as if we at the power plant were totally cut off from the world. 'Fancy meeting you here,' people would joke, and the atmosphere lightened. We still had to go back to the control room later, but now we were all committed so it was nothing special anymore. On the other hand, having been relieved of the burden of protecting the 'non-combatants' who would have had to suffer with us for no useful purpose, now, all of us were in the same boat. We were the ones who were going to fight to the end. There was no feeling of desperation. In fact, it was almost exhilarating!"

Yoshida and his team had by no means given up. On the contrary, they felt less burdened now and their morale rose. It was the beginning of a new campaign.

"We knew what we had to do. Collecting the data from the plant was the duty-team's job, while the fire-fighting squad and the recovery team were responsible for injecting water into the reactor. Then there was the job of restoring power, and refueling the fire engines. If we could keep all those going, we could stop things from getting worse. And under those conditions we had to go back to the reactor. We hadn't stayed to just die. We were there because we had a job to do."

Everyone was physically run down by now. All the toilets in the QPB were crimson.

Izawa recalled, "The toilets were in a terrible state. There was no water to flush them. We'd brought in portable toilets and when they were full we'd carried in more. It was an endless cycle erecting them, and they were filled with blood. Everyone was passing blood. Late in March, we got the water running again but the urinals themselves were stained red for good. We were all on our last legs."

Now that those six hundred people had been evacuated from the building, the total left was just sixty-nine. In the hostile environment, these men, who the foreign media later came to call the Fukushima Fifty, pressed steadily on with the work they had in front of them.

The contractor

Conflict of interest

Day 5—March 15 Evening

"Somebody help me! Can anyone drive a truck? We need someone who can drive a fire engine."

Twenty kilometers from FDI, Mari Satō's voice rang through the darkness in the gymnasium at the Fukushima Daini nuclear power plant. The only lamp was at the entrance. Its feeble light barely illuminated the figure of Mari Satō, of the Disaster Prevention and Safety Group, standing with a megaphone in hand. She was at her wits' end and almost in tears.

Yoshirō Abé of the Niigata office of "Gembō" (the Japan Nuclear Security System) thought: *That's a job for me. I can do that.* He was one of the contractors who, immediately after the earthquake, had come all the way from Kashiwazaki to offer support at FDI. Gembō is a security company established in 1977 to provide security systems, primarily for nuclear facilities.

Abé, however, was a veteran fireman who had spent thirty-seven years at fire stations in Niigata prefecture. He had joined Gembō at the age of sixty and, as the requirement was for fire-service experience rather than security expertise, had been dispatched with two younger employees to assist with the water supply, arriving at FDI early in the morning after the earthquake. They had started water supply operations along with another contractor, Nam-mei Industries, and had worked around the clock until Site Superintendent Yoshida had sent them to take shelter at FDN on the morning of March 15. Incidentally, three of the Nam-mei employees were injured in the hydrogen explosions at Units 1 and 3.

Now Mari Satō stood before them at the gymnasium at FDN, yelling through her tears.

"Help! We've got to find someone. Isn't there anyone who can help?" she called frantically. Only that morning, leaving Yoshida and his sixty-eight men sitting, as if for ritual suicide, to face their deaths, she and the rest of the six hundred non-essential TEPCO employees and contractors' staff had retired from the quakeproof building at FDI.

Now they were accommodated in the gymnasium at FDN. But there was a limit even to the determined efforts of the sixty-nine. In particular, as time passed, the shortage of people working on water injection at the reactors began to tell.

"It couldn't be helped. The work was simply too much for the limited number of people left at the plant. That's why, little by little, some of the people who had earlier retreated to FDN began to return to FDI. They were going back into highly radioactive areas, so they must have had misgivings," pondered Satō.

"At times like this people reveal different sides of their character. I mean, everyone has family to think of and their own burdens to bear. But in the afternoon, people from each group began to make their way back to FDI.

"The people at the reactors had somehow held things together, but they were sure to need more hands. Some groups left it to the individual. Others went back because they were asked to. The people from the fire-fighting squads went back, too. But the mental conflict was hard. One of the young men asked me to let him think about it. He sat there for about half an hour leaning back against the wall of the gym with his head in his hands. His children were still small," she explained.

"The torment, the conflict – it was painful even for us watching. There were those who had made up their minds and were impatient to go, and they'd keep asking him if he'd made up his mind yet, if he was going or not. He'd beg them to wait a minute and hide his face again. I felt really sorry for him. I really learned a lot about human nature during all this – the things under the surface of people on the edge. It was really painful to watch. That young man sat there deliberating for half an hour, by the way, but he finally decided to join his group and head back to the plant. It must have been agony for him."

It was amidst all that torment that Satō, now crying herself, was yelling for assistance. It must have been the heroic effort put into her appeal that pricked Abé into action. He had already spent three days at the plant on the water injection operation, so he in particular must have been more aware than most of the predicament at the reactors.

"Satō-*san* was in the dark gym, frantically pleading for help. Some of the fire engines got wrecked in the explosions, so they simply didn't have enough of them at the plant. They sent out an appeal for more, and several were supposed to arrive somewhere nearby. But the drivers didn't bring them into the plant where they were needed. To make a long story short, they were scared of the radiation, so they just parked the fire engines and left. Somebody had to go out and drive them to the plant, connect them to the water supply and all the rest of it. The trucks were all 'fire engines,' but they were from different manufacturers, so they were operated differently. It was pretty complicated. And they were short of people, too. By the time Satō had finished shouting "Isn't there anyone who can help?" into her loudspeaker, she was crying. Anyone with a heavy vehicle license could drive a fire engine to the plant, but there was more to do than that. And that limited the number of people who could actually help."

And one of them, of course, was Abé: a veteran with thirty-seven years' experience employed in fire stations, he was an expert in the field. Not only could he drive, but he was confident he could handle anything that might come up while using fire engines in the reactor injection. He'd go and help them. He made up his mind. But it was not to be so simple.

"We worked for a contractor, not for TEPCO, so we had our own boss whose orders we had to follow. The boss in Tokyo said he couldn't allow his employees to go into such danger, and forbade us from going into the plant. Well, I could understand his feelings, but . . ."

The veteran fireman

Day 5—March 15 Overnight

Just at that moment, Satō had taken her microphone and called "Mr Abé of Gembō, Mr Abé of Gembō, there is a call for you. Would you come over here, please?"

There was a call for him on the only cellphone that could get through to the ERC. Abé, who had been in the farthest corner of the gym, hurriedly picked his way between the people lying on the dark gym floor to where Satō stood.

"It's from Mr Abé," she said.

This was Takanori Abé, the head of the Disaster Prevention and Safety Group, who just happened to have the same surname.

"Mr Abé, the engine of one of the fire trucks has stopped again. Would you mind telling us how to refill the water tank?"

"To refill the tank, you first had to lift the hose out of the water and let the water drain out of the pump. And there were a number of other steps to the procedure.

"Group leader Abé said he was about to do it himself, and wanted me to teach him how. But that's a tricky job to do alone. There's the location to think of for a start, it's pretty heavy, and then someone needs to operate the pump. It certainly wasn't something an inexperienced person could manage alone. When I heard the situation I suddenly felt pathetically powerless. I actually started crying. I really wanted to go the plant and help him, but . . ."

In his mind he saw the group leader struggling alone in the darkness. It was so gut wrenching he simply burst into tears.

"If the water doesn't go up the pipe properly you have to do the whole thing over again, you see? Just thinking of him having to go through all that just made me feel so sorry for him I couldn't stop myself from crying. I even said I'd go and do it for him. But I'd got the chairman telling me not to go, and, as a company employee, I couldn't go against a direct order. And there was no way to get in touch with my boss to ask him directly. And he was an old TEPCO man, too. Anyway, I told him (the other Abé) I'd go if I could get permission. Also I asked if he could try to get my boss to agree by calling him directly."

Seeing Abé crying in front of her, Satō felt grateful, she says.

"Mr Abé from Gembō was on the cellphone with tears pouring down his face. I really wanted him to go and help, but he was a contractor employee, and contractor employees aren't allowed to make that sort of decision by themselves. As he stood there with tears running down his face, I felt really grateful for what he said, though."

After a while, they managed to get in touch with the chairman of Gembō, but his primary concern was preserving the lives of his employees. He was worried that if he made an exception for Abé, there would be another and another, until he ended up with a large part of his staff back at the plant. Despite the fact that the Japanese term for these contractors means 'co-operating industries', he didn't feel they were obliged to co-operate as closely as that. He told Abé that he'd have to grin and bear it.

Using the unreliable cellphone, Abé repeatedly guided the Abé at the plant through the procedure, and then, on the morning of the sixteenth, the boss gave his permission.

"I suppose we've got to do what we can," he said, finally approving the weeping Abé's request.

"Abé," he said, "Sorry about all this. You will go, now, won't you?"

Though the chairman had been concerned only for his employees' safety, Abé's enthusiasm had swayed him.

"Yes, sir! Sorry to have troubled you, sir. Thank you very much!"

Abé was finally allowed to return to the plant at FDI. Though he was heading into danger, his heart was full of gratitude.

"The chairman was worried about me getting killed, so I guess it was an uncomfortable decision for him. But I was really delighted to get the go-ahead. During the night I'd had numerous discussions with Abé-*san* at the plant. In one of them he told me he wanted to use the fire-hose to pump water thirty meters into the air and direct it into the building, and wanted to know if this was possible. It depends on the pressure, of course, but the effective vertical reach is normally only twenty-five or perhaps twenty-seven meters. If it's within that range we can do it, I told him. But it would be best if I could go and help run things. So once I got permission to go, there was nothing I could say but *Thank you.*"

Backup

Later, Abé from Gembō learned that while this was going on, a support team from Kashiwazaki had reached the nearby city of Iwaki.

"I used to be an instructor for the Gembō fire crews at Kashiwazaki, and three of them in their mid-twenties had heard that we'd gone on ahead and imagined we must be having a hard time.

So they'd volunteered to come and back us up, and had got as far as Iwaki, I heard. When they got to the office in Iwaki, they had been asked why they'd come all the way from Kashiwazaki at a time like this, and had been told off for being reckless. They'd replied that their advance party had got into difficulties, so they had come to back them up. The Gembō staff in Fukushima were astonished. If we'd come all the way from Kashiwazaki, they couldn't sit around and do nothing, they realized. They had to help, they said. And they'd tried to come all the way to the plant. But I didn't hear anything about all that until afterwards. Even though they were only contractor's people, they were really keen to help."

Abé left Gembō six months after the disaster, at the end of September 2011, and is now enjoying his retirement.

"I sometimes go for a drink with the lads who went to Fukushima that time; the three of us who went first and the other three who came later. 'That was quite a trip, that was!' we'd recall. Personally, I'm really glad we had some stout-hearted lads like that. Good people to work with. You know they'll keep going when it comes to the crunch. I've always had a kind of principle that I'd always try and do better than other companies. So I was tickled pink that, they pulled out all the stops to come and back us up, even in the middle of all that. When I heard that there were some younger lads who thought of us as mates and came all that way to help us out, I knew they must be really good guys."

With life and death in the balance, the focus continually swung from one disaster to another. At one moment the radiation peaked, only to fall again while instead the pressure in the reactor suddenly spiked, mocking the efforts of the men at the reactors, before suddenly falling again.

There weren't many who would go willingly into that kind of situation.

"We were so isolated, as if we were in another dimension," recalled Mari Satō. "There were things we needed desperately but none came. It was so quiet there, a peculiar kind of hush. Actually, a lot of the supplies we needed had already been shipped to the coal depot at Onahama, but some things had been taken back while others were left in strange places. It was a crazy situation."

The battle at the reactors was far from over. They struggled on.

The military: Do or die!

Helicopters and lead suits

Day 6—March 16 **Morning**

During the sixteenth of March, the plant personnel who'd retreated to the safety of FDN poured back into FDI.

"We've got to keep the water going in!"

This task, which Yoshida had stressed from the start, required manpower. So the people who were needed at the reactors flowed back from their temporary shelter.

The work of keeping the water flowing was proving to be a cat and mouse game. They would work like mad to keep the reactor from getting out of control and then it would sit there quietly for a few hours only to flare up again, and then the process would be repeated.

The reactors weren't the only cause for concern. Beside each reactor stood a pool of water containing spent fuel rods. It was feared that the pools next to reactor Units 3 and 4, which had earlier suffered explosions, might have been damaged by the blast or by falling debris. If the water from the pools were lost, these fuel rods too could melt down. With the roofs blown off the reactor buildings, the pools of spent fuel rods were open to the sky, which meant that if the fuel there melted down the radiation released would be enormous, and the effects incalculable. These pools needed to be hosed to keep them filled with water.

While the activity at the plant continued in its own isolated dimension, TEPCO decided, again, to call on the military for help. That afternoon, Toshimi Kitazawa, the Minister of Defense, sent instructions to General Ryōichi Oriki, his Chief of Staff, to send helicopters to drop water on the plant.

As soon as they could, the huge CH-47 Chinook helicopters lifted off for Fukushima, while three more helicopters were sent to monitor the radiation around the site. On this day, however, the radiation was literally off the scale, so the day's operations were postponed.

During the monitoring flight, it was noticed that there was water in the pool at Unit 4, but as there was steam rising from Unit 3, there was a strong probability that the water level there had dropped, so it was decided to give priority to cooling Unit 3.

So now, the Ground Self-Defense Force was fighting its campaign both on the ground and in the air.

The units thrown into this operation were from the JGSDF 1st Transportation Helicopter Group, based at Camp Kisarazu in Chiba. (See map page vi.) Immediately after the earthquake, Flight IV of the 104th Flight Squadron, under Lieutenant Colonel Kenji Katō, had moved to Camp Kasuminome, an airfield near Sendai, and had been providing support and supplies to the earthquake and tsunami disaster area. Just before nine in the morning of March seventeenth, the CH-47s with Katō aboard, took off bound for Fukushima Daiichi. The first helicopter, manned by Kato and four of his men, followed by the second with another four men aboard, picked up its cargo of water from the sea off Sendai and headed south for FDI.

The container used was a device known as the Bambi Bucket. Two point two meters in diameter and two point four meters tall, it could be dipped into the sea to automatically fill with up to seven point four tons of water.

The fore-and-aft twin rotor Boeing CH-47 Chinook helicopter in its camouflage paint has been in use since it appeared during the Vietnam War in 1962, not only with American and Japanese forces, but also in Britain, Australia and Taiwan. It is a large transport aircraft, essential for mobile military campaigns, and the most popular such aircraft the world.

"So this is the place, is it?" said Lieutenant Colonel Katō, thirty minutes after takeoff.

As they gradually drew near the FDI site, the only thing on his mind was how he was going to carry out his mission. Of course this was the first time he'd seen the plant directly since the accident. Katō scanned the view ahead over the shoulders of the two pilots, forty-year-old Major Teruki Itō and thirty-two-year-old First Lieutenant Yoshiyuki Yamaoka. He'd flown nearby on numerous training exercises so, even though he'd never flown directly over the plant, it was a familiar sight.

"Wow, so those are the reactors."

Today, for the first time, the special nature of this mission made him consciously examine the plant.

"Just before we arrived, they had been monitoring the radiation and had discovered that the levels weren't much lower than the day before. I told my crew and the other helicopter that we would go ahead as planned, but instead of hovering thirty meters above the building while we made a stationary drop, we'd drop the water as we made a pass at ninety meters. Then I had to think about how to release the water exactly onto the target."

Depending on the radiation levels, the water could be dropped while the helicopter hovered over the target, but since the levels were just as high as the previous day, he decided to make a moving drop. Of course, a stationary drop was more accurate, and would put more water on the target, but with the radiation levels over the reactor so high, the danger was too great.

The atmosphere among the crew was different from their usual flight exercises. The radiation worry was one thing, but the thing that really changed the mood was their protective gear. Under their flight helmets they were wearing full-face masks, while over their normal flying suits they wore lead-lined reconnaissance suits. These included a lead collar to protect the thyroid glands in the neck.

All this protection made them very conscious of both the danger and the importance of their mission.

"What surprised me was the weight. It must have weighed about twenty kilos, so it really dragged you down. There was lead in the collars around our necks and even in the gloves. The collar was held in place with a bit of Velcro, but we gave up on the gloves and used our normal rubber ones. The lead ones were so cumbersome we couldn't have operated the switches."

"We weren't overly concerned about the radiation. Generally speaking, the bits that need protecting are the internal organs. We'd used the protective masks before, so they weren't a worry either. But we did have a problem in that we couldn't hear each other. It's usually so noisy in the cockpit that you can't hear if you speak normally, so we have lip-mikes inside our helmets. With them we can usually hear each other just fine, but with the protective masks on, of course, the lip-mikes couldn't reach our mouths. We had to tape the mikes to the holes where our voices came out of the masks."

Katō's machine turned to starboard from its southerly course over the Pacific. From above, with its roof blown off, the reactor building looked like a ruin. But Katō was too immersed in completing his mission to be moved by the desolation of the scene.

"There was no roof on the building, only steel girders, and there was all kinds of debris strewn around. Seeing it up close, I was appalled at the damage."

Something else that worried them was the tall exhaust stacks around the building. If a gust of wind were to carry the helicopter even slightly off course, it could collide with one of them. They had to be especially careful.

"The reading on the digital radiation meters we were wearing rose as we approached. Once we got this far, there was nothing more for me to do. The pilot would give the sign, and the mechanics behind us would press the switch."

The two mechanics were forty-year-old Sergeant Major Tsutomu Kimura and thirty-one-year-old Sergeant Kenji Nakajima. Katō was located right between the mechanics and the pilots. Just as in their usual drops on forest fires, the sequence of operations was already fixed.

Unit 3 was right ahead of them. Tension rose as their altitude fell.

"Ready! Releeeeease — — NOW!"

As Katō gave the command, both Kimura and Nakajima pressed the button. The black lever on its cord has a red button at the tip. Kimura and Nakajima pressed it together, and the water poured out.

"As we passed overhead, the radiation picked up by the meter spiked. It must have been pretty hot. The switch is usually operated by one man, but Kimura and Nakajima said they pressed it together. I guess they wanted to be sure. I had my eyes on the target the whole time."

The drop was over and the mechanic yelled over the noise to confirm, "Drop complete. No problems."

"*Ryōkai!*"

It was 09:48 when Katō commanded the second machine to follow suit.

"Chopper 1, finished. Chopper 2, go ahead!"

Chopper 2 acknowledged. Katō's machine left the area for the meantime and refilled the bucket from the sea directly off the plant. They were going to make another drop.

Five minutes after Katō's machine, the second helicopter made its drop, and at 09:56, Katō's machine made its second. At 10:00 the second helicopter finished its second drop, and the two machines left the site, continuing south to land at J-Village, twenty kilometers away.

J-Village, which straddles the boundary of the towns of Hirono and Naraha, was built as the first national training center in Japanese soccer history. During the Japan-Korea FIFA World Cup of 2002, the top seed, Argentina, made J-Village its official training camp.

As the home ground of the TEPCO women's soccer team 'Mareeze', and, just twenty kilometers from FDI (as well as being next door to TEPCO's Hirono thermal power plant), it was now running fulltime as a center for disaster recovery operations.

"We landed on the soccer pitch nearest the sea. Unlike many of Japan's soccer fields, it was a real turf pitch. The monitoring chopper had landed ahead of us; we came down near it and the second machine followed us in. We were told to hold our positions there. It took ages for them to check the radiation on the outside of the machine. We turned off the engines and just sat there waiting in our lead suits. After that, they worked out how much radiation we'd actually been exposed to and told us it was equivalent to having just a few X-rays, so there was nothing to worry about. All the TEPCO people as well as the JGSDF personnel were wearing those white protective suits."

Though they had made two passes directly over the reactor and the radiation had spiked each time, the short time spent in the danger zone and the heavy protective suits had kept them from harm.

Katō was from Shiogama in Miyagi Prefecture, Fukushima's northern neighbor, with a daughter in sixth grade and a son in fourth. That day, his daughter was due to graduate from elementary school.

"My family knows that when there is a disaster of some sort, I'll be away from home for a while. This just happened to be the day of my daughter's graduation ceremony. Of course I knew that, but during the mission I forgot all about it. While I was away on this mission, I only managed to get through once on my mobile. It was only long enough to ask 'Are you all OK there?' For the rest of the time, I was totally absorbed in the mission and the graduation never entered my mind. It wasn't until the evening of the day after the water drop was completed that we managed to get through by e-mail and I told them that all was well at my end. My wife wrote back, 'Don't worry. We're all fine here. Go and get the job done.' She knew when she married an officer that there would be times when I'd be sent to the front."

Crash tenders

Day 6—March 16 Near midnight

The water-drop wasn't the only mission given to the Self-Defense Forces. Joint Chief of Staff General Oriki sent orders to the other forces, too, to support the fire brigade's operations on land.

"Send two fire engines and six personnel to FDI to assist with hosing the reactors."

The orders reached forty-year-old Lieutenant General Toshiaki Matsui, commander of the Air Civil Engineering Group at JASDF Hyakuri Airbase, in the town of Omitama, Ibaraki prefecture, at around midnight on the night of March sixteenth.

To put it simply, the Air Civil Engineering Group is the unit responsible for the management and maintenance of the base. Also, in case of fire, they are provided with their own fire engines.

"I'd already heard about the hydrogen explosions at Fukushima Daiichi and about the awful situation up there from the news on TV. But until then I hadn't imagined we'd end up going there ourselves," Matsui recalled.

"I guess it must have been on the fifteenth or sixteenth that, from different sources, the idea that they might need our fire engines reached me. JASDF bases are normally equipped with two fire engines. The seating is arranged so that crews can quickly get suited up while the truck is in motion, and has a variety of gear aboard at all times, so you'd imagine there was plenty of space, but actually it's not quite as simple as that. After we received our orders, three of us got into each vehicle and set off. There are two rows of seats, so we sat with two in front and one behind. I couldn't honestly say we weren't worried about radiation, but our orders were to prepare and leave immediately, so I remember we were more concerned about getting our stuff together and getting on the road as soon as we could, than about the risks."

They left on the morning of March seventeenth at around 03:30, but not before borrowing radiation dosimeters from the medics, who explained that if the alarm went off they had to retreat.

"We put on the dosimeters and set off. Fire engines are pretty slow, so we didn't reach the Yotsukura parking area on the Jōban expressway near Iwaki, about fifty kilometers south of FDI, until around seven or eight in the morning. It must have taken four or five hours. There were several JGSDF fire engines there already. There was a JGSDF Lieutenant Colonel in charge there who told us we were to leave immediately and assemble at J-Village before heading to FDI together. When we left for J-Village it was our airport crash tender that was selected for the mission. Above the seating compartment there is a roof-mounted turret equipped with a powerful water cannon. These air-force crash tenders from JASDF can pour six tons of water onto a target in just one minute and have a range of eighty meters. This kind of machine made possible a totally different method of cooling from the one used so far, that of linking hoses to pump seawater for injection into the reactors.

"The fire engines of the normal type, which could only spray with ordinary handheld hoses, were to be held in reserve at J-Village. I decided to take forty-three-year-old Master-Sergeant Katsuya Harada and set off in the lead in the AMB3 airport crash tender, which can carry ten tons of water."

Even once they reached J-Village, the order to proceed to FDI didn't come through. Matsui and Harada waited for hours in their protective white Tyvek suits and goggled masks, and when they finally set off for FDI, it was past 16:00 in the afternoon and the sky was beginning to darken.

"We were given no explanation for why we'd been kept waiting there so long, so I've no idea what was going on. We didn't feel particularly desperate, though. We were already formed up in convoy and it took us a couple of hours. I'd heard it was about an hour by car, but fire engines are not exactly sports cars, and travelling in convoy slowed us down too, so it seemed to take forever."

Also in the convoy was thirty-nine-year-old Sergeant 1st Class Yūshi Saitō who had come all the way from Camp Kisarazu, in Chiba, with the fire and rescue squad of the Headquarters Service Company.

"We formed up at Yotsukura and drove on to J-Village before heading for FDI. The main reason it took so long was the dark. The TEPCO people who were supposed to guide us knew where the cracks and bumps in the road were, and where the tricky parts were, and so they zipped ahead, but we couldn't keep up," he said.

As the darkness deepened, their feeling of insecurity on the unfamiliar road grew.

"For one thing, the fire engines' water tanks were fully loaded. Some of the bridges had been damaged by the earthquake and might not able to support the weight of our trucks. So, we'd have to stop and wait while each truck crossed, one by one, and that took up a lot of time. We'd be guiding each other, checking as we went, like: 'This bit's OK' or 'You can get through over here', and the like; but one by one we brought the trucks through.

"Worries? Yeah, the radiation was a worry. I mean, we'd already been given iodine tablets to take, way back at Yotsukura. I think we were all worried about it. What with the fact we were wearing our CBRN reconnaissance outfits, and that the iodine tablets we'd taken were supposed to protect our thyroids, there was obviously good reason to worry. So, yes, we were worried."

Saitō's ground forces' fire engine followed Matsui's air force machine through the night toward Fukushima Daiichi.

Hosing Unit 3

Day 7—March 17 18:30

By the time the convoy reached the main gate at FDI it was already 18:30. Matsui's air force crash tender and the ground force's fire engine with Saitō aboard had arrived.

Matsui and the other senior officers went inside the security building beside the entrance. There they received detailed instructions from the TEPCO staff about the work they were to carry out. A map of the site was laid out in front of them.

"We'd like you to hose down the reactor known as Unit 3. Rather than go directly to Unit 3, we'd like you first to assemble at a point between here and there, and then go to the reactor one vehicle at a time."

It was already completely dark outside. Once inside the security building, everyone took off their goggles. They had electric power in the building. Under the fluorescent lights, Matsui could feel the tense mood among the TEPCO personnel as they explained the situation.

"The TEPCO people who explained things to us were quite young. We were to proceed to the midpoint between the entrance and the Unit 3 reactor, and then go from there to hose down the reactor in turn. When one vehicle came back the other could go, water the reactor and come back in turn, he told us."

The orientation took all of thirty minutes.

Matsui and the other self-defense force personnel made their own decision on the order of their turns. They decided to send the GSDF's CBRN (Chemical, Biological, Radiological and Nuclear) reconnaissance vehicle first. They decided that this vehicle would go to the reactor and get up-to-date radiation readings, and, if the readings were above the expected levels, the vehicle would return with red lights flashing and with its loudspeakers blasting the signal to retreat.

The meeting ended as the TEPCO employee announced, "Now, let me escort you to the site."

"During the orientation, I wasn't scared; I was more worried whether we'd be able to follow our instructions correctly and actually find the Unit 3 reactor. I mean for starters, we'd never been there before; and on top of that, it was already completely dark. The guide from TEPCO said he'd lead us to the reactor, but to be strictly accurate, we had to go one vehicle at a time on the road from the assembly point midway to Unit 3, so from there on, it was like, *I'll wait for you at the end of the road*! Well, we just had to follow the road, so it shouldn't be too difficult, but you know how things go. . . ."

At last, Matsui and his men had started work. As arranged, the GSDF's CBRN reconnaissance vehicle went first.

It's a special reconnaissance vehicle capable of sampling and evaluating the environment even in radioactively contaminated areas. This vehicle went down to the reactor site. When it came back, Matsui's crash tender would go next. After a while, the reconnaissance vehicle came back. Its red lights weren't flashing and neither were its loudspeakers blaring the signal to retreat. It was the go-sign.

"Ours was the first fire engine to go," recounted Matsui. "We lurched our way down the S-shaped curves in the dark. It wasn't terribly steep. The dosimeters that the medical squad had issued us with before we left the base were rod-shaped. Under our Tyvek suits we were wearing our GSDF combat gear, and the dosimeters were in the breast pockets. We got down the slope and had just reached a kind of crossroads just before Units 2 and 3, when suddenly my alarm went off."

Pip-pip-pip-pip-pip went the artificial sound. In fact both of them went off together, surprising Matsui. But with dosimeters being in the pockets of their uniforms under their Tyvek suits, they couldn't see what the actual readings were.

"Sir, the alarms have gone off. What shall we do?" asked Sergeant Harada.

When they'd left their base, they'd been told that if the alarm went off they had to retreat, Harada reminded him. But at the moment something caught Matsui's eye.

There was someone standing there!

It wasn't completely dark here. There were several lights powered by generators like those used at construction sites. It had been pitch dark all the way down the slope, but here there was light. And there was someone standing there in a Tyvek suit. He was waving them to come forward.

Before them, the Unit 3 building loomed eerily. Their alarms continued their pipping, while outside there stood a man directing them and their crash tender.

"I was amazed," recalled Matsui. "I don't want to give the wrong impression, but it was awesome to see a man actually standing out there in all that. It was inspiring to see that the people on the site were so incredibly dedicated, and it made me forget all about the instructions to retreat if the alarm went off. I went ahead and gave Sergeant Harada his orders.

"Let her rip!"

"Yes, sir!" Harada replied, moving the truck forward and beginning to operate the control levers for the turret. Harada was in the driver's seat with Matsui in the passenger seat. It was about fifty meters to the target, but with a maximum range of eighty meters, that distance was no problem.

To measure the distance accurately he sent a short ranging burst. The TEPCO man, who was standing directly ahead of them, signaled: *A bit more over that way.*

Harada rotated the turret a little to the right. He'd been slightly off target. The man outside raised his arms to make a circle over his head: *OK!*

Harada pressed the button firmly. The machine roared. A blast of water shot out toward the target – ten tons of water in a little over two minutes. The noise was frightening.

The pair of them, Lieutenant General Matsui in the passenger seat and Sergeant Harada in the driving seat, just sat and gazed wordlessly at the jet of water. In what seemed like no time at all, the ten tons of water were gone into the reactor building.

"The man outside gave us another OK sign. *We did it!* I thought. It was a great relief being able to live up to the hopes pinned on us. I was delighted!"

Their alarms were still *pip-pip-pip-ping* away. The noise didn't stop until they'd left the vicinity of the reactors. They did a U-turn and returned up the slope to the assembly point, having fulfilled their mission and feeling well satisfied.

"Nice work!" Matsui called to Harada.

"Thank you, sir," he replied. With their goggled masks on, it was hard both to speak and to hear, and the conversation ended there.

After they got back to J-Village, Harada asked, taking off his mask, "Did you forget, sir?"

"Forget what?" asked Matsui, puzzled.

"The bit about retreating if the alarm went off, like the medics told us," explained Harada. *Oh, yes!* remembered Matsui. He realized that the moment he saw the TEPCO man standing outside it had been wiped from his mind.

"Afterwards, people asked if the radiation levels weren't high, but we were inside the fire truck, and there was a guy there standing out in the open. I don't know if preoccupied is quite the right word for it, but we were certainly determined to deliver the water as ordered. Once you're on the job, you get absorbed, and that's what keeps you going. We simply had to live up to what was expected of us. There was also the fact that we were amateurs as far as radiation was concerned, and we didn't know enough about it to be too scared of it. There was a bit of that to it, too. And that TEPCO guy there. He was wearing a mask so we couldn't tell who he was, and he was standing out there in all that. . . ."

Matsui's work ended with this one sortie. On the following day, the eighteenth, a different crew manned the same vehicle. On the twentieth and twenty-first, the ground, air and maritime self-defense forces each participated in a total of three sorties, sending a total of five loads of water onto the target.

Matsui returned to his home base at Hyakuri on the nineteenth.

"That was when I got in touch with my family," Matsui recalls. He had a wife, a son in eighth grade and two daughters in seventh and third grades.

"As I'd expected, my wife complained that I hadn't told her I was going. I made some excuse about forgetting because we were in such a rush. The children too asked me if I had really gone to FDI. 'Sure did!' I told them. They were glad that I'd got back safely but I didn't tell them the details."

Here was another father who had gone to the front and faced death.

It worked!

Day 7—March 17

So, where were GSDF Sergeant Saitō and his fire engine from Kisarazu during all this?

On the seventeenth and eighteenth he was busy with the hosing operation. On the first day he had followed Matsui and Harada in their air force crash tender, and had unloaded his tank of water into the reactor building.

"We went in turns, each one setting off as the previous one came back. It was a simple matter of following the one road, and the first time, I thought it was just an ordinary hill, but next day we went down in daylight and saw that it was really quite steep. It was a kind of meandering lane, not straight at all. At night, we only saw the bits lit up by the headlights, so we had no idea what it was really like. When we got to the bottom of the slope there was a TEPCO man to guide us, so we stopped to have a word with him."

Saitō's fire engine was a B2-Class machine, with searchlight and loudspeakers, which they used to communicate with the guide.

"We used the searchlight to pinpoint what we thought was the target, and when I used the speakers to ask the guide if we were on target, he gave us the OK sign, so we opened fire."

Unlike the air force fire-fighting squad, the ground forces crews actually use the word "Fire!" when they let loose with the turret water cannon. It comes more naturally to people used to using artillery. So Saitō called "Fire!" and water shot into the air.

"At Unit 3 there was a rectangular hole in the wall. It must have been blown out by the explosion. That was what we aimed for. I made two trips; the first time, we aimed for that hole, and the second time, I remember we shot further back," Saitō recalled. "Sure, we all cared about our own lives, but when you've come to do a job like that, the first thing on your mind is accomplishing the mission. Whether or not your own life is in danger is the last thing on your mind. We were told we were going there to cool the reactor, so I had an image of filling some pool with water for cooling it down later. All we'd been told was that we would put water in the fuel rod pool and they'd use the water to cool it down to prevent a meltdown."

Saitō recalled that other units beside the GSDF had come to help, too, and that it had been a race against time.

"We were well aware that we had to get there as soon as possible; minutes were precious. All we could think of was that if we didn't deliver loads and loads of water as quick as we could and get the temperature down, it would be all over. In fact, once we started, we found it took less than three minutes to discharge a full load. The next vehicle would be waiting behind us, so we were very conscious that we had to vacate the space and let them get to it as quickly as we could. And even once we finished the job and got back, there was still the worry whether we'd actually made any difference."

Saitō didn't get to hear about how effective their work had been until he got back to the J-Village.

"When we'd finished spraying, we were really concerned whether what we'd done had been any use, whether we'd done enough. At that point we didn't know what effect it had had. When we got back to the J-Village, we heard for the first time that the temperature in the reactor had dropped. The officer who'd been in charge of the cooling operation at the plant that day came around and told us that as a result of our mission the temperature had fallen. When we went back the next day, they told us they'd keep us up to date on what effect we were having, and we arranged to go again if the water level dropped. It was really encouraging to hear that our effort had done some good."

When the Self Defense Forces weren't at it, the plant's own fire-fighting squad and recovery groups, under the command of Site Superintendent Yoshida, were busy, endlessly supplying water to reactors 1, 2 and 3. It was a task that required enormous tenacity. In that isolated dimension at FDI, with the assistance of the Self Defense Forces, the cooling operation plodded on. It was a sign that the runaway plant was at last beginning to yield to human persistence.

Family

You're alive!

Day 8, March 18

Why are they crying? she wondered.

In the midst of the unending struggle at the plant, Mari Satō of FDI's Disaster Prevention and Safety Group was puzzled at the weeping voices of her family at the other end of the phone. Reflecting on it now, she suspects that under the extreme conditions at the plant, she may have lost some of her own capacity for emotion.

It must have been March eighteenth, she remembers. It was a whole week after the earthquake, but it was the first time she had been in touch with them since the disaster.

"You're alive!"

Her husband, her twenty-two year old son and nineteen year old daughter at the other end of the line, were speechless to find that their wife and mother, whom they had feared dead for a week, was still alive.

It was hardly surprising. On TV they had seen the awful scenes of the tsunami and of the damage wrought by the hydrogen explosions at the plant.

For two days, three days, four days and soon a week, there had been no word from Mari. Forced to evacuate themselves, they had given her up for dead.

And then suddenly, there she was, on the phone.

"I no longer had my own mobile, and I didn't have the children's numbers in my head. On top of that, there were hardly any working phones in the building, so there was no means of getting in touch anyway," Mari recalled.

"The earthquake happened during the spring break, so both the children were home from college, and I heard later that after the quake they'd taken their grandparents and evacuated on foot. Eventually they all ended up at my son's digs in Tokyo. Then, a week later, I was able to borrow a cellphone from the head of my group and managed, via the TEPCO HQ communication center, to call my son's phone at a number that I'd found hidden away in a corner of my address book. I was really lucky and got through. I was so frustrated with everything that was going on that I didn't feel sad or anything. And there they were crying."

On learning that Mari was alive, their tears welled up.

"Hello?"

"Huh? Mom?"

"Yes, it's me."

Her son yelled to the others, "It's Mom. She's alive!"

Their mother, who for a week they had thought was dead, was there on the line. The young man's voice cracked with surprise and joy. The three of them took turns on the phone. The father started with "You're alive!" and gasping through his tears immediately asked "Where are you now?"

"At work, of course. In what we call the QPB."

"What are you doing there?" her husband continued. "I thought you must have been killed in one of the explosions. We were expecting the next time we saw you would be laid up in hospital, or the morgue!"

Satō had no idea of what was going on outside the plant. It was hard to imagine.

"It hadn't occurred to them that I might still be at work. They had talked about it and decided they might be able to find me at a hospital somewhere or more likely in the morgue, they said. They'd seen the explosions and couldn't imagine I'd survived. Knowing me and my job, they thought, I'd probably been out there manning a fire-hose and had got caught in the blast, they said. And they couldn't stop crying. My husband was choking on his words. But I was already pretty much out of my mind and couldn't understand what they were thinking. I'd already gone past that level. I guess most of the people who'd been with me in the plant were the same. We were so – what's the word? Frustrated? Stressed out? Shell-shocked? Anyway, we were past crying. We'd already repeatedly been through situations where we thought the end had come, so I couldn't understand why the family were all crying on the end of the phone. Looking back on it now, it's hard to understand myself at that point."

You would expect that someone who'd been through the continual extreme stress to which Mari had been subjected would be ready to drop, but in fact she felt frighteningly fit.

"None of us had been getting enough sleep, but somehow I felt perfectly calm, and in peculiarly good shape. We had a TV in the night duty room, and it happened to be on at the time, and just by chance we happened to be watching a press conference in which someone from the national Fire and Disaster Management Agency who had returned to Tokyo after visiting the plant was weepily describing the horrors at a press conference. It was a peculiar feeling to watch it, considering that there were still hundreds more of us here at the plant. I guess we'd gone past the normal human limits and all kinds of feelings were going numb. I can't remember how long it took to get back to normal again."

In fact, it wasn't until five months later that Satō actually broke into tears.

"Gradually, I started to remember things and go over things that had happened. The first time I really cried, it must have been August. As part of the recovery work, I had to drive through deserted towns like Kawauchi, all kinds of places, and there were dead cows lying around, foxes coming out, all skin and bones they were. I went quite often and once a fox cautiously crept up to me. 'With a tail like that, you must be a fox,' I said to it, and got out of the car to give it some *ampan* (a bun filled with sweet bean paste) that I happened to have with me. It looked so skinny and miserable, I just suddenly, out of the blue, burst into tears. Not only the people, the poor animals, who had done nothing to deserve it, were in a terrible state, and we'd done this to the whole area. Even the animals were suffering. The cows got skinnier until their bones stuck out. They gave birth to calves, but those just died. It was terribly sad. Seeing living creatures afflicted like this, I started to comprehend the damage that had been inflicted on the human population, and then the tears came."

It was seeing the non-human suffering, the innocent animals, that triggered her feelings for the human victims.

"When I saw the scrawny, starving creatures, I felt so sorry for them, and angry at what we humans had done to them, and then the tears just wouldn't stop," explained the unshakable Mari Satō.

Saying "Thank you"

Day 3—March 13 In retrospect

After people have survived life-threatening situations, they frequently recall things that they have left undone.

When forty-eight-year-old Kazuhiro Yoshida, the supervisor from Units 5 and 6 who volunteered to make a second attempt on the failed vent, realized there was one thing he had left undone, he became depressed. The matter that troubled him was his family.

"When I got back from the control room to the QPB on March 13, it occurred to me that I had left all sorts of things unfinished," he said. "The big one was my family. I have a daughter at college and a son in high school. The daughter is away at college in Tokyo, so there were just the three of us living at home in Futaba. My wife and son just happened to be at home when the earthquake struck. It was my day off and I'd just come home after a day out, so I thought I'd better go to the plant. I'd been out in my own car, but after the earthquake, the traffic jams were so bad I'd abandoned the car and run home. The house isn't far from the plant, so I went to check the damage at the house, and when I went to have a look around outside, there was an emergency broadcast over Futaba's town-wide speaker system, from which I learned that there had been some catastrophic event that fell under Article 10 of the Nuclear Emergency Act."

Yoshida had been with his family soon after the earthquake. He had no idea that the situation would subsequently go downhill, and when he left the house he hadn't said any particular words of farewell.

"I knew I had to go back to the plant, but also guessed that there would soon be an order to evacuate. I was thinking that I'd have to take them to the evacuation shelter when the order was actually given. I'd already abandoned my car in town, so I took the two of them with a change of clothes, our bankbooks and *hanko* (the official seals used in place of signatures), and dropped them off at the evacuation shelter."

Then he drove to work in his wife's car. After that he was completely occupied risking his life. While he was busy on his volunteer mission amid intense radiation to try and vent the Unit 1 reactor, his family vanished from his mind.

He didn't even think about them again until he was relieved from his shift at the control room and arrived back at the QPB on March 13. Then, after all that he had gone through – the explosion in the Unit 1 reactor building, the vent, and all the rest of it – he was suddenly worried sick about his family.

When he'd delivered them to the evacuation shelter, he'd made sure they had a mobile phone and recharger, and had given them instructions on using it.

"With these power cuts, there's no telling when you'll be able to recharge it again, so keep it switched off, and only switch it on when you have to use it. You'd better keep in touch occasionally, when you need to."

But he had no idea what had happened to his wife and son since then. The evacuation zone had kept expanding, and then the reactor building had exploded, and there was no longer any way to check up on them.

Even at the ERC in the QPB, they had no information about the situation in the immediate area. Yoshida was getting frantic because of something he'd left undone.

"I got in touch with my wife from a company computer," he recounted.

"The machines in the ERC can send e-mail to the outside, so I used one to e-mail my wife's mobile, and luckily it got through."

He asked her to let him know simply where they were, and what their situation was, and told her that there was a crisis at the plant. That e-mail reached his wife but there was more that he had left unsaid.

"I hadn't thanked her. By now, I didn't think I'd get home alive. The TV was on in the ERC, so I expected that my family would know how bad things were at the plant. I wrote a little about that, and then added something like *Thank you for everything. We had some good times.*"

With the plant in its current situation, Yoshida was thinking about the possibility of his dying. If he died without seeing them again, that parting at the evacuation shelter would be their last. It would be such a pity if that were the last memory they had of him, he thought. He had very much wanted to leave them, especially his wife, a few more words of gratitude. Looking back, he remembers distinctly how, when it occurred to him that he hadn't done so, he felt heartbroken and became extremely depressed. In that e-mail, he wrote briefly about the aftermath of his death.

You mustn't complain to the company, he wrote. It was quickly becoming his last will and testament.

"Strictly speaking, I didn't think that I was definitely going to die; only that it was a possibility. I didn't go so far as to say I *wouldn't* be back. But, *We had some good times* effectively meant I wouldn't be coming home. *Look after the kids,* I wrote, too, I seem to remember. Sending her a few words of thanks, that last thing left undone, took a huge weight off my shoulders."

Having once retreated to the ERC, Yoshida and the others could now go back to the front line in the control room with their determination renewed.

The question of whether we can really leave anything for our families left behind must be of immense importance to men about to risk their lives.

The reply that Yoshida received was a distillation of the love of his whole family: *Don't be silly. You have to come home. Now!*

Izawa's family

Shift supervisor Ikuo Izawa, head of the Unit 1 and 2 control room, often found his head full of scenes from the place where he grew up. It was like part of his family to him.

Since early on, Izawa had promised himself he would stay at the plant to the very end. He was resigned to dying there.

"I knew I had to stay there and send the others back, decontaminated and alive. To do that, I'd have to remain in the control room. I didn't know how the end would come, but I knew I wouldn't see my family again. I hadn't been in touch with them. There was no way. But, yes, I thought about them a lot," he recalled.

"What first made me think about them was when we had to actually go and carry out the vent, and that kind of job. All the people in the surrounding area had had to evacuate, so when I thought about the scale of the disaster, I knew this was our last option. We had to do everything we could and then somebody would have to stay behind and see it through, and I realized I was the only one for that job. That was when I really thought about my family."

Didn't he feel he had to tell his wife and family of his plans?

"She knew I was the shift supervisor that day and I'm sure she understood what would happen if a situation like this came up. She knew that I'd have to stay to the end whatever happened, so there was no need for me to tell her so directly. On the other hand, the situation out there was getting really serious, so I was more concerned that *they* should stay safe. That was when I visualized them."

For the last five years or so, Izawa's wife had been confined to a wheelchair by her worsening rheumatism. His mother had passed away long before and his father, born in 1926, now lived with them, so Izawa must have been at least slightly concerned about his family.

"I was worried about my wife in particular because she's disabled. Whenever I'm away overnight on duty, she stays over at a care-center. While I was busy dealing with the accident, I would have liked to ask my sons to take over the responsibility of looking after their grandpa and their mother, but there was no point fretting about it, since there was no way to get in touch. So, once I'd got used to the idea that I was never going to leave the control room, I had too much to get on with right there in front of me to have time to worry about the family."

The burden that a family constitutes is different for everyone. When Site Superintendent Yoshida gave the order to evacuate all but the essential staff, Izawa, for the first time, sent an e-mail from the ERC to his three sons, the oldest aged twenty-six:

It looks as if I'm going to have to stay here for good, so I need you boys to look after your grumpy Grandpa and your moaning Mom for as long as they need you.

He tried to squeeze a bit of humor into this declaration of his commitment. But one son replied *What are you on about, Dad? You'd better not die on us.*

"My youngest boy, he's only nineteen, mailed back *No way! I'm having a drink with you again someday.* Cheeky under-age brat, I thought. Typical boys. Can't string more than three words together."

However short they may have been, the messages conveyed the respect and love they had for their father.

"Later, I learned that when the explosions occurred, my wife was still at the care-center. When she heard that they were going to have to evacuate because of the Unit 1 explosion, her hands shook, she told me. I guess she was afraid something might have happened to me. At this point, the family were all split up, evacuated by the military and the care-center's vehicles, to hospitals and evacuation shelters, and I heard that the boys and other relatives spent two weeks going around them all before they located and were finally able to go and pick up their mother."

Did Izawa ever get to see his home again?

"The evacuees were occasionally allowed to go back to see their homes, and I went back several times. My old home was actually still standing and not even badly damaged. It was just as we'd left it except for the weeds that had sprung up all around it. The earthquake had covered the roads with fissures and the ancestral gravestones had all fallen over. It was pretty bad."

The family graves were on a small hillock about five hundred meters from the house, in a graveyard shared with several local families.

"When winter came and we were allowed to go a second time, I went to see the graves. The first time I went back, we were restricted to a limited area because the grass and bushes might still be contaminated with radioactivity, so I wasn't able to visit the graveyard. The second time we were allowed along the road, but not into the undergrowth, so I could only see the graveyard from a distance. I could vaguely see what looked like my family's graves poking out of all the weeds and bushes. I come from quite an old family so there were about three monuments there. But the gravestones had all fallen over in the earthquake and lay hidden in the grass. All the old stones seemed to have fallen down. I think my dad was pretty upset that he couldn't visit the graves."

His wife still hasn't visited the house, he said.

"She's stuck in a wheelchair, so she hasn't been back to the house yet. Next time we're allowed back in I plan to take her with me, but she says she'll stay in the car, so she'll just look from there without going indoors. She wants to take another look, too, so I'll take her with me next time."

As both an operator at the FDI plant and a victim of the disaster, Izawa has a better understanding than anyone of the scale of the damage that the nuclear power plant project has brought to the area. Knowing the suffering of the local people, time will not relieve the weight on his shoulders.

The missing technician

An unexpected phone call

It was on a Sunday in late August of 2012 that I visited the small city of Mutsu, in the corner of the Aomori's hatchet-shaped Shimokita Peninsula. It was my first visit there in twenty-eight years. (See map page vi.)

My previous visit there had been in 1984, as a journalist for the editorial section of a magazine, on an assignment that, coincidentally, related to nuclear power. After the port of Ōminato had been selected as the home port for the nuclear-powered research ship *Mutsu*, there had been conflict between the pro- and anti-nuclear factions, which I was there to cover.

The refreshing blue of Mutsu Bay was unchanged.

This time, I was here to visit a family in an attractive bungalow on the outskirts of town. They were the parents of the late Yoshiki Terashima who had died, aged twenty-one, when the tsunami struck the basement of the turbine building at the Unit 4 reactor at FDI.

After the earthquake, Yoshiki Terashima of the Operation Management Department at FDI had gone with a colleague to inspect the basement of the Unit 4 turbine building, only to be overtaken by the tsunami. Their bodies were not recovered until March thirtieth, almost three weeks later.

He and Kazuhito Kokubo were the two engineers at the plant whose young lives were taken by the unforeseen tsunami.

I had come north to Mutsu to offer incense and prayers for this precious life sacrificed in the execution of his assigned duties, and to interview his parents.

This couple who had lost their twenty-one-year-old son were

still young themselves. The father, Kazuyuki, was forty-seven and his wife, Yuriko, forty-five. Kazuyuki, a government employee, had at the time of the quake been posted, alone, to far-off Wakkanai, at the northernmost tip of the north island, Hokkaido. I had come to hear from them with my own ears about the loss of their son and how they had taken this unforeseen nuclear disaster.

I had made an appointment, so the Terashimas were waiting for me at their cheerful, white, sunlit, two-storied home.

The earthquake had severely shaken Mutsu, four hundred kilometers away in Aomori prefecture.

Yuriko had been indoors at the time. Yoshiki's two younger siblings were a sister in eleventh grade and a brother who had just graduated from junior high school and was about to start senior high.

"The ground shook slowly, side to side, like this. My son was home, since it was the spring holiday, and a couple of his friends had come around. The quake was like nothing I'd felt before, and the boys and I all went outside. When the shaking eventually stopped, we went indoors again. Just as we got settled down, the shaking started again. The first time had been pretty big, so the electricity was already out. Just as we headed outdoors again, my son noticed a kind of clicking sound. With the power cut off, the phone couldn't ring the bell as it normally did, but made this noise instead. I noticed the sound but didn't realize what it was, but my son understood and picked up the receiver. I was wondering why he didn't come outside, and went back to the living room to see where he was. He was talking on the phone."

"What's the matter?" she asked him.

"It's Yoshiki," he answered.

"Yoshiki? Why?"

She took the phone and heard Yoshiki's voice.

"Yoshiki?" she inquired, and, in a perfectly ordinary voice he answered, "Are you all right, there?"

"Yes, we're fine. The power's out but we're OK."

As she spoke she began to wonder. Because of the power cut, Yuriko had no source of news from outside, and because of the size of the tremors, she'd assumed the epicenter must have been nearby.

But the fact that her son was calling from four hundred kilometers away in Fukushima must mean that the earthquake had been felt there too. So she asked him.

"How are things there?"

Yoshiki had joined TEPCO in April 2008 and had been posted to the Fukushima Daiichi plant. There had been quite a few earthquakes in the nearby Sendai area, so each time, they had been sure to keep in touch.

The nature of his work made both mother and son sensitive to the risk from earthquakes. Every time there was an earthquake, they'd send e-mails or phone.

"Things shook a bit, but we're fine," her son answered. Now she knew that Fukushima had been affected too. Not only Aomori, but Fukushima too had been hit four-hundred kilometers away. It must have been quite a big one.

"The electricity went out right away here. Do you have power?" Yuriko asked.

"Oh, yes," he replied. This was before the tsunami. The plant was still powered by its own emergency diesel generators.

"Oh, that's good. You don't need to worry about us here either," she told him, and he seemed relieved.

"OK, 'bye, then," he answered cheerfully and hung up. He was more concerned about his family than his own safety. Of course his mother could not have foreseen that these would be the last words she heard from him.

"We checked up on each other every time there was an earthquake. He always used to tell me how he was run off his feet after every earthquake with all the extra checks that had to be carried out. Actually, the previous day we'd heard that his little brother had passed his senior high entrance exam, so I'd sent Yoshiki an e-mail and in the evening he had phoned. We must have talked for nearly an hour. At New Year, all five of us had been home, for a change, so we'd had a long chat then, but I don't think we'd had another chance since then."

Having heard from her son that he was safe and well, she felt reassured. It wasn't until the following day, March 12, that circumstances changed.

"It was a phone call from my mother in Hokkaido, that changed everything," Yuriko told me.

"I grew up in Hokkaido, and my mother called me from there

on the twelfth. She'd heard from a friend who'd seen on TV that people were missing at TEPCO, and who thought she'd seen Yoshiki's name on a list that scrolled across the screen. They had electricity in Hokkaido but we were still cut off, so we hadn't heard anything at all about the tsunami. We didn't even know what news there was out there concerning the earthquake. I'd already called my mother and told her that I'd had a phone call from Yoshiki right after the earthquake and that he was fine. She already knew that, so I thought she was getting soft in the head or something, and told her that he'd called me the day before, so how could he possibly be missing? But before I finished talking to her, a neighbor of mine who'd known Yoshiki since he was tiny came around to the house to speak to me directly."

The neighbor's news was a bombshell for Yuriko.

"I didn't hear it myself, but on the radio they said that TEPCO employee Yoshiki Terashima, age 21, is reported missing."

On hearing that, Yuriko lost her composure. She'd already hung up the call from her mother, so she immediately called her husband in Wakkanai.

Yoshiki's father, Kazuyuki, recalled: "I was away in Wakkanai at the time and had seen the news on TV. I knew about the tsunami. It was a shock, but I knew Yoshiki had been on the phone to my wife, and I know how robust the nuclear plant buildings are, so it never occurred to me that he might be in danger.

"That must have been about eleven on the morning of the twelfth, so as soon as I got the call from Yuriko, I called the TEPCO head office in Tokyo and they told me they were unable to contact him at the moment so he was listed as missing. *In that case, why hadn't they let us know directly?* I complained. Anyway, I knew I had to get back home, so I got in the car and drove the ten hours from Wakkanai to Mutsu. I got in touch with TEPCO head office several times but they were all mixed up and didn't know what was going on!"

They were getting nowhere talking to head office, so they got in the car and went to speak to the people at TEPCO's construction office on the coast in Higashidōri.

Yoshiki had graduated from Mutsu Technical High School and had been taken on to work at the nuclear plant that was being built at Higashidōri, and was currently in training at FDI. For this reason, the people who had been involved with Yoshiki's entrance examination were at the TEPCO construction office. Yuriko told the story.

"We got in touch with the people at TEPCO HQ, but they had no idea what was going on, so my husband and I decided to go directly to the office in Higashidōri. Kazuyuki phoned them first but they didn't even know that Yoshiki was missing. They knew there were people missing at FDI, but the fact that one of them was from Mutsu hadn't got through to them."

This says a lot about the muddle at TEPCO. The Terashimas decided to get the Higashidōri construction office there to contact TEPCO HQ directly, and slowly information started to filter through.

"One of the Higashidōri people brought us a plan of the FDI plant and explained all about it. They showed us where they thought Yoshiki might have been at the time of the tsunami."

But at the same time, the information put an end to any hope of finding their son alive. The news was exactly what they didn't want to hear.

"After that, the water continued to pour in, they said, but it couldn't drain out again, and then they began to discover all the contamination, too. We asked them why they didn't go and find him sooner, why they couldn't find him right away, but they told us the basement was in a terrible state. The amount of water was amazing. It seems that there was a lot more water in Unit 4 than the other reactors."

Their son had been sent into danger to carry out an inspection, had he? They could imagine him battling on in the darkness to fulfill his mission.

It would be just like him. Where others might hang back, he'd press ahead and do what he had to do. That was how they'd brought him up, they recollected.

But the thought that it had cost him his life was to be a long-lasting burden for them.

The ideal son

Yoshiki Terashima was born in 1989 at his mother Yuriko's parents' hometown of Otobé on the Japan Sea coast of Hokkaidō. When he was three years old, they moved from Mutsu to Matsumaé in Hokkaido when his father was posted there, returning to Mutsu when Yoshiki started third grade. He stayed in Mutsu through the rest of elementary school and high school, growing up in the severe but stimulating natural environment of the Shimokita peninsula.

"Yoshiki was too good for us. He was such a good boy you wouldn't believe he was brought up by ordinary parents like us. He was naturally kind to people. He never showed off, but just carried on diligently, never caused us any worry or got into trouble. He was always very good like that."

Yuriko told me how he had looked after his younger brother and sister, and was never insolent to his parents. That was Yoshiki for you.

"He was such a thoughtful boy. We had the two younger ones to look after, so he used to think for himself and make sure he wasn't a burden on anyone, even when he was little. He never threw tantrums – a really gentle big brother – and he didn't go through the usual rebellious teen stage either."

For the Terashimas, Yoshiki was a son to be proud of. His father, Kazuyuki, who was frequently posted to distant parts for long periods, said he thought the fact that Yoshiki had developed into such an admirable son had something to do with his own absence.

"I'm not often at home, usually," he explained, "so he always realized that he had to be careful not to be a burden on his mother. Even if something came up, he was the oldest, so it was like he'd suck it all up and not show anything. He had a way like that. He was always trying to make sure we never had to worry about him. He was very tough that way."

This rare kind of boy that you don't often see these days – one who could take whatever came – eventually grew up into a man. He joined the judo club in junior high school and belonged to the rowing club when he went on to Mutsu Technical High School. The school had won the national championship at one time and maintained a national level team, and Yoshiki, even after injuring his back, stayed active to the end.

There was a certificate of his still displayed in the living room where his parents talked with me. At Mutsu Tech he had passed his national examinations and gained qualifications in numerous subjects, and this was his Junior Meister Gold certificate, awarded only to those who achieve a total score of over forty-five points.

The Junior Meister system was started in 2001, with the objective of sending out into society students with specialist skills, knowledge and qualifications. Gold is, of course, the highest of the levels awarded.

Each qualification earns the holder a number of points. For example, Electrician First Class counts for a certain number of points, while Second Class is worth less, with points awarded according to the difficulty. Yoshiki had amassed a considerable number of qualifications during his time as a student, and reached the level of Junior Meister Gold.

"In his second year at senior high, Yoshiki won a prize for his efforts in arts and sciences. Getting his qualifications was important, but he also had to keep his school grades up, and he coninued practicing hard with the rowing club, too, so it must have been a really tough two-and-a-half years. Sometimes when he got home from club practice it was about nine o'clock, so there wasn't much time left for homework. When there are tests coming up, the clubs are supposed to take a few days off, but if there's a competition coming up, they don't. I asked Yoshiki when he got his homework done, and he said he used the breaks at school. He was a serious, diligent lad. I guess he must have spent every free moment studying."

It is by no means easy to get a job in a huge company like TEPCO, but Yoshiki got a good recommendation from his school and was one of only two from Mutsu Tech who passed the demanding TEPCO entrance exam that year.

Besides examination results, the entrance test also takes into consideration the applicant's attitude and character, so maybe it's not surprising Yoshiki was chosen.

"It's different every year, but normally only one or two students from Mutsu Tech get into TEPCO. First they get weeded out at school. There were two in Yoshiki's year. I think, when they made the selection, the school also took into account the fact that he'd stayed three years in the rowing club at the same time as getting all those qualifications. He was taken on to become one of the mechanical staff at the Higashidōri plant once it was complete. So, then he was sent off to plants in Niigata and Fukushima to study and gain some experience so he could come back and work at the new plant here in a few more years. . . ."

Kazuyuki still lamented the loss of his son's future.

Seven thousand cranes

Late March

This life of indefinite waiting was unbearable for the family. A week, ten days, two weeks, time passed but there was no news of Yoshiki. *With all the advancements of this modern world, why couldn't anyone find him even though they knew where he must be? The fire brigade had rescue units: Why couldn't they go and find him?*

The couple fretted over the delay, unable to comprehend the obstacle presented by the fierce radioactive contamination.

Kazuyuki recalled their frustration.

"I thought they could simply send divers in there and find him. But there was so much guesswork going on we were getting nowhere with the facts. With only two men missing, why couldn't they go and look for them? The office in Higashidōri tried to find out for us, too. As time went by, however much we wanted to keep our hopes up, the reality was that the odds of finding him were getting worse and worse. We began to entertain the thought that he might not have survived. There wasn't much progress on March 28 or 29 either. Until he was found, everything was just suspended."

Kazuyuki even went so far as to ask them to allow him to go to the site himself.

"I forget exactly when it was, but they told us that what with the earthquake damage and all, they had all sorts of things that had to be done and didn't have enough people to spare for a search. I told them I thought searching for the missing people came first in my book. That was how it started. They said that today a search had been carried out but they hadn't found him, so I asked where they'd searched, but they didn't know. There's no use in telling us something like that; but that was how it went on. I can do scuba diving, so I offered to go and search myself. That's how frustrated we were getting."

In the midst of all this, a cruel rumor that the missing two had run away from the plant started circulating on the internet. Somebody claimed to have seen them out for a drink in Kōriyama.

In consequence, the wife of the other victim was reported to be suffering from shock. All of this came in the midst of a whole wave of TEPCO-bashing.

"It went so far that someone on a TV program said that they should catch jerks like that and string them up. We had already lost hope, but of course we still wanted them back alive. We, his parents, knew better than anyone that Yoshiki would never abandon his post. We were appalled to hear stories like that."

On the other hand, they'd have been delighted to find that he really had escaped alive, said Kazuyuki. But Yoshiki wasn't the kind of person who'd do that.

To keep her sanity through the hellish days, Yuriko began to fold paper cranes. She'd started on March 12, when they learned that their son was missing.

"There's nothing else we can do. Let's make some cranes," suggested Yuriko to her daughter. Yoshiki's sister went to the same Mutsu Technical High School. With her mother, who had lost her will to do anything, Yoshiki's sister started folding origami cranes for her kind older brother.

These tangible prayers for Yoshiki's safety grew in number.

The school heard about it and other people started to help making cranes. It was near the end of the final term of the school year. There were still a number of teachers at the school who had been there in Yoshiki's time. None of them was likely to have forgotten that diligent student who had gone on to work at TEPCO.

"The teachers helped too, even using lesson time to fold cranes together, they told me, while some students made more at home and brought them in. I started because I couldn't set my hand to anything useful, and then everyone started to help. The number of cranes grew. Looking at the ones people had made for us, I found some that were beautifully folded and some that weren't; there was quite a mix. But that just proved to me how they were all trying so hard to help. I was so happy to realize that everyone was praying for Yoshiki's safety. It was such a support to know they were all behind us. Without that I don't know how we'd have got through it."

There were already seven thousand cranes. As the cranes were delivered, the Terashimas threaded them all together, counting as they went. When they reached seven thousand, there was a phone call from TEPCO.

"We've found a body which could be your son's."

It was nearing the end of March.

"Ever since Yoshiki had gone missing, my husband had been on leave from work. Because of the situation with our son, the company kindly decided to treat his time off as 'standby duty'. But the days went by without any news, and the next day and the next. It was getting so long that my husband said he felt he had at least to go and show his face at the office, and so he went back to Wakkanai. And the day he got back, a message came for him that Yoshiki had been found."

At that point, it was just a single line saying that a body had been discovered.

"The water level in the basement had dropped a little and, though they couldn't recover it, they could see what looked like a body, the message said. They said they would go back the next day to recover it. The water level had dropped but it was still waist deep, but they had managed to get in there by boat."

At the coffin

At last they'd found him. Their beloved son was dead. Yuriko recalled the curious feeling she had at the time.

"I hadn't thought for a moment that Yoshiki wouldn't be coming back. It wasn't a possibility I'd even considered. I didn't care what state he was in as long as we could bring him home to Mutsu. I sort of skipped over the matter of whether he was alive or dead. I just couldn't accept that he was dead. I must have been completely off my head. The thing that I was most afraid of was the possibility he'd been carried off by the sea. I didn't mind what state he was in, I just wanted to bring him home. That was the only thing that concerned me – whether we could bring him home."

When they got the news, the first thing she thought was that now they could bring him home. She'd been so concerned that he might have been washed away by the tsunami that it transcended the matter of life and death. Looking back on it now, she finds her own behavior quite incomprehensible.

The whole family made their way to the plant.

"Yoshiki had been in a cold, cold place for so long, we took blankets with us to Fukushima, as well as the origami cranes," she explained.

The place where they were to see their horribly disfigured son again was TEPCO's Hirono thermal power plant, twenty-eight kilometers south of FDI. The family members were shown to a place like a prefab site office. Inside were two rooms, each containing the coffin of one of the men who'd been missing.

According to the account they heard, Yoshiki's body had been found floating in the water, while the other had been left by the retreating waters, four meters up on a piece of machinery.

They were warned, "His injuries are pretty horrible. Do you really want to look? I don't think it's advisable." This was partly the result of the three weeks it had taken to discover them. Nevertheless, the coffin was opened. The body was inside a zippered plastic bag.

The coffin was the kind where the face could be seen, but the head had been covered in bandages and couldn't be seen directly. One of the TEPCO staff asked Mr Terashima if he would like to confirm the identity directly.

"We have some photographs you can look at instead."

Rather than oblige them to inspect the body directly, they had printed out photos from the autopsy.

"I had a look," said Kazuyuki, "and thought the others shouldn't see them. His face was recognizable. There were pictures of his face, his torso, and close ups of some of the badly damaged parts. There's no doubt the face was Yoshiki. After I'd looked, my son and daughter had a look at the photographs they had printed out."

Yuriko flicked her eyes over the photos but couldn't bear to look at them directly. The face looked somewhat swollen.

That was enough for them. It was definitely Yoshiki.

"Yoshiki, we're here. We've all come to take you home. You must have waited for ages. Let's go home to Mutsu now." Yuriko wrung out the words. "It was such a long wait, wasn't it. You can rest now."

This son who had never been any trouble to them whatsoever now lay silent in the coffin. He'd tried so hard at everything; he'd been so kind and he had doted on his parents; and now he slept, wordless. The days since he had been born rewound through Yuriko's head.

"Yoshiki, you did well," his father murmured. "Well done, son."

At his side, the brother and sister he had always taken care of took it all in silence.

"At that moment, the main thing was that we had found him," recalled their father, Kazuyuki. "The others were able to accept that their big brother had worked to the end and had died doing his job. He hadn't tried to desert his post. He wouldn't do something like that. The other children seemed to accept that, or so it seemed. Personally, I couldn't help being proud that he had tried so hard. When they went down into the basement for the inspection they'd discovered a leak in the pump room. They'd reported it back and were working out how to fix it when the phone was cut off. That's the scene that I imagined as I looked at the photos of the body."

When the bodies were discovered, neither was wearing a helmet or safety harness, he was told.

Their helmets could easily have been knocked off by the impact of the water but the safety harness has complicated hooks and could only have been removed deliberately. The fact that they had both taken them off means they must have had a few seconds after the water started to come in when they realized they were in trouble. I can imagine the two of them might unconsciously take them off to get rid of the weight and escape more easily."

The autopsies showed they hadn't drowned, but had died of shock due to multiple external trauma. It was thought they had died from being thrown around by the force of the inflowing water.

"Because they were in the basement, we'd assumed they must have drowned. We couldn't imagine how they could have died of shock down in the basement. But when we got the details we realized that the manholes and the like had been open, because the building was undergoing scheduled maintenance, so the water must have gushed in all at once. That's what we thought must have happened. The body was absolutely covered in bruises and marks where things had hit it. All kinds of bruises, and the legs had multiple fractures, they said."

Yuriko recalled: "The Unit 4 reactor building is the one nearest the sea, I heard. And because they were doing an inspection, the shutters, which are usually closed, were all open, and the manhole covers were off, too. So when the tsunami first came crashing in, there were lots of places for the water to get in – many more than usual. It was an awful lot of water."

The bodies clearly explained how the first rush of water pouring in must have killed them on the spot.

Departure

April 3

Yoshiki's body came home to Mutsu with his family on April third in the coffin accompanied by the origami cranes. In fact, it was buried in them. The cranes folded to wish for Yoshiki's safe return now covered him completely, and under their protection, Yoshiki returned to Mutsu in Aomori prefecture.

For Yoshiki, it was the first time he'd been home since the New Year holiday.

Unlike most of Japan, in Mutsu, it is the custom to have the cremation *before* the wake. Until then, Yoshiki spent the time alone with his family. Before the wake, they went to the crematorium, with the coffin still enveloped in the wreaths of origami.

Then, Yoshiki's body was consigned to the flames accompanied by the seven thousand paper cranes.

"It was as if the thousands of cranes would fly him to heaven," said his mother.

Surrounded by those seven thousand paper cranes, Yoshiki Terashima set off on his last journey.

More than three hundred people gathered for the funeral. His classmates and many more who had admired him in life for his diligence and gentleness attended.

"Lots of students from his grade, other people with connections to the school, and many of the people who'd played a role in Yoshiki's life attended. His contemporaries from senior high had spread out all over the country, but they went to the effort of coming back from far away. Even the classmates of his siblings came. They said they were so shocked they couldn't stay away. I guess the just couldn't get over it. Even afterwards, old school friends came around to pay their respects by offering incense and prayers, and we'd have a chat, and I felt that many of them seemed unable to accept it all – the scale of the accident and the fact that Yoshiki was involved, and the way he died. It was all too much," explained Yuriko appreciatively.

Later still, colleagues from Fukushima came to pay their respects, a few at a time, until the total reached a matter of dozens. Each of them had their own story to add, and the Terashimas gradually began to grasp the whole story.

Yoshiki's father, Kazuyuki, filled me in on what they learned.

"When the earthquake came, Yoshiki first evacuated his section from the building and then set off to the basement to inspect the damage. During the evacuation there were about eight people together and because it had been such a huge earthquake everyone wanted to phone their families. Apparently, the only ones who managed to get through were the two who died. Then an alarm or something went off, and orders were issued, so Yoshiki had to go and get on with his inspection. He and his partner went down to the pump room in the basement and discovered there was a leak there, and then reported that back to their boss, so I'm sure he carried out his responsibilities right to the end."

Yuriko spoke tearfully of the colleagues who took the trouble to travel all the way to Mutsu.

"His workmates told me how there had been so much to do getting things straight after the earthquake, and how they'd slaved every day hoping to find the missing pair. We hadn't realized how hard they'd tried, searching for them every day, determined to find them with their own hands. I was so grateful for their efforts."

While she had been folding paper cranes to help keep her sanity, her son's workmates had had their noses to the grindstone trying to restore function at the plant, she learned.

"They came all that way just to talk to me about Yoshiki. I was really impressed with the solidarity among the employees at the plant. It was hard for us, but for them it must have been terrible; one of their own had disappeared right in their midst, but they had to keep working. I could understand their pain. They'd taken the trouble to come all this way, so I was really glad to find out what nice people Yoshiki had been working with."

Yoshida, the man

Yoshida surprises his wife

Day 7—March 17, Tokyo

"Hello? It's me!"

"Papa? You're alive? Are you all right?" Yoshida's fifty-five-year-old wife Yōko answered, incredulous at the sound of her husband's voice.

You're alive? Yes, that was probably the most appropriate thing to say in the circumstances. Until he phoned the family home in Tokyo, the atmosphere there had been despondent, as the matter of greatest concern for the family of Masao Yoshida, Site Superintendent at the Fukushima Daiichi nuclear power plant, was whether he was dead or alive. Almost a week had passed since the earthquake. The reactors had started to cool, but it was still too early for complacence. Yoshida, who had at last got around to thinking that he should let his family know he was still alive, managed to get through to his home using the cellphone which had finally started working again, and a connection via the TEPCO HQ communications network.

The news that the mass media brought from the plant had been of hydrogen explosions and rising pressure in the reactors, which merely served to emphasize the precarious situation at the plant. For his family, the news on TV about the grave situation at FDI was directly tied to their father's life. When his wife asked if he was still alive, he'd answered, "So far. I'm still here."

This was typical of him. He didn't make a fuss about things, but neither did he make little of something serious. He continued, "I don't know how things will turn out, but that can't be helped.

Anyway, I thought I'd better let you know I'm alive at the moment."

With subordinates all around him, it was no place for the Site Superintendent to be having an intimate chat with his family.

"The 'old lady' wasn't crying then, you know. I guess she didn't have the strength for it right then," Yoshida explained. "I asked her about it later, but she said it was just one thing after another. First, the place where her husband was working was hit by an earthquake, and then by a tsunami. That alone caused a huge fuss. Then Unit 1 blew up, and then Unit 3 blew up too, and she saw all these sensational scenes on TV. It was worse than anything she could imagine, all these things one after the other. She was past crying."

Yōko herself recalled, "The news coming out was just so horrendous, there's a kind of gap in my memory. I had a sudden phone call from my middle son telling me to turn on the TV at once, and as soon as I did, the first thing I saw was the reactor building explosion. My mind simply went blank. I hadn't a clue what to do and I just sat there watching the TV. All I could do was pray that my husband was safe."

The couple had three sons, aged thirty, twenty-seven and twenty-four. From then on, Yōko spent day after day with nothing to do but fear for her husband's life. It was more than a month before he was able to take three days leave and come home.

"I think it was in April, when he finally managed to get home for the first time after the accident. It wasn't until I opened the door of our apartment and saw his face that I really believed he had come back alive," she said.

On his return from the living hell of the accident, Yoshida looked haggard. He had lost weight and grown a beard.

"One look told you how much he'd been through, but what really surprised me was the way he was dressed. He was wearing these really gaudy pajama things. Training wear, I think they were. And he'd come all the way home from Fukushima dressed like a clown. All his other clothes had been thrown out because they were contaminated, and he was dressed in things that looked as if they'd come from the thrift shop. But I was so happy to see him home that I burst into tears."

He was only allowed two nights at home. Though the cooling

operation at the plant was proceeding steadily, it wouldn't do to have the commander absent from his post any longer than that.

The day after his return to Tokyo saw his wife bawling her heart out. She was convinced her husband had committed suicide, she told me.

"The next day, my husband said something about everything being on his desk and disappeared out of the door. After he'd gone, I went and looked at his desk and found his wallet, the bankbooks, his mobile phone and the like, all neatly lined up on his desk. Seeing it all like that I thought: *Surely not?* I mean, lining up the bankbooks like that and then leaving, it was a weird thing to do. It worried me sick, and I even thought he might be going to do something stupid. I'm from Shizuoka prefecture, and I phoned my older sister who lives there to ask her what I should do. She'd got a good grasp on what kind of man Masao was, and assured me he wasn't the kind of person to do something foolish. I managed to calm down, but it was still an awful worry."

Her husband had been through a frightful experience, and in addition had lost two of his young men. It wouldn't be so surprising if his mind took an unusual turn after he managed to escape from the torture of life at the plant. The anxiety grew in her like a balloon.

"I was so anxious I thought I'd burst. Then, about an hour later, the front door creaked open and as if nothing had happened he called out 'I'm home!' I was speechless. Immediately, I clung to him, and started to cry like a baby. I *never* cry out loud. I don't think I'd cried like that since I was tiny."

Yoshida himself was astonished. "What's the matter?" he asked. All he'd done was slip a little cash into his pocket and go around the corner for a haircut. Hair gets contaminated by radioactivity very easily, so he'd wanted to get his cut as short as possible.

"He's a big man, so there I was clinging to his waist, crying my eyes out and he hadn't a clue what was going on. He just stood there with a silly grin on his face asking 'What's the matter?' When I told him I thought he'd gone out to end it all, he said I should know he wouldn't do anything like that. It had suddenly occurred to me that he might have wanted to try to take responsibility for everything by taking his life. When he came back safely, my balloon just burst."

In retrospect, it was clear that Yoshida wasn't the kind of man to do something like that. Ever since he was young he'd always kept a copy of Dōgen's *Shōbō Genzō,* a thirteenth-century Zen Buddhist text, at hand. He'd even taken it with him to his office in the quakeproof building at FDI after the earthquake.

One of Yoshida's hobbies was visiting temples, and he was always thinking about life and death. It makes you wonder if it was fate that sent her husband to handle the disaster.

Bodhisattvas

Masao Yoshida was born in Ōsaka and attended Ōsaka Education University's junior and senior high schools in Tennōji before proceeding to the Tokyo Institute of Technology. At junior and senior high he was a member of the kendo club. He was the only child of the owner of a small advertising company.

"I got to know Yoshida when I joined the kendo club at senior high," recalled Professor Masanori Baba, Vice-Dean of Kagoshima University's Graduate School of Medical and Dental Sciences, "but at first I didn't realize he was in the same grade. I thought he was one of the seniors."

"The kendo club didn't have its own dojo, you know, so we used to practice in the gym. When I joined, I noticed this tall, skinny boy, who seemed to know his way around. I guessed he was one of the seniors. It was the first time I'd tried kendo, and when he said to me 'Hey, you! You've never done this before, have you?' I had to admit it, and then we got chatting. I found out we were in the same grade and we started hanging out together."

Professor Baba talks of Yoshida as a man with an aesthetic.

"How should I put it?" he pondered. "Even in senior high, Yoshida was a man with his own aesthetic, a certain path that he wouldn't stray from. If he decided on something, he'd be sure to carry it through. That aesthetic was the way he lived. When we had a kendo camp, if I griped about something, he'd tell me off like an older brother. He never complained himself; he had his own internal standards and objectives. It wasn't only the kendo club, either. He loved physics, so he formed a physics club, and a folk-song club, too. He was very conscientious about consideration for others and friendships. A kind of Kensaku Morita character. Exuberant, but with a talent for caring.

"Yoshida went straight to Titech after finishing high school. I didn't. It took me an extra *rōnin* year to get into the college of my choice. While I was an unattached *rōnin* I lived in Osaka. Yoshida was worried about how I was getting on and wrote several letters to encourage me. I still have them at my parents' house. I guess Yoshida thought I might be feeling depressed. And he couldn't just leave me to get on with it. He was the only one who wrote to me to buck me up like that. No one else did. We met up once in my *rōnin* year. 'I was worried about you,' he said. 'But you look much better than I expected. I don't know why I bothered to come.' That's the kind of big-hearted guy he was."

Hiromichi Sugiura, the head priest at a temple in Nara, spent the eleventh and twelfth grades in the same class as Yoshida. He retains a strong impression of him.

"Both of us were cheerful and exuberant boys, I remember. He wasn't one to fret over the small stuff. I guess there was some religious education behind his attitude. I think it was in eleventh grade that he asked me if I knew the Heart Sutra. My father was head priest of a Buddhist temple, but at the time I didn't want anything to do with that kind of stuff. I hadn't learned any of the prayers and sutras, and then, out of the blue, Yoshida says to me 'Sugiura, your family runs a temple. You really ought to learn at least that one,' and there and then he starts to teach me the Heart Sutra. He knew it by heart, and recited it straight off. Quite a surprise, that was. From an eleventh grader at that. Even at that age he had an interest in religious stuff."

Sugiura recalled this episode because of a video he'd seen on the internet. Yoshida had made a video appearance at a symposium in Fukushima city in August 2012, seventeen months after the disaster. In it, Yoshida had spoken of seeing his employees flocking back into FDI and how they had reminded him of a famous passage in the Lotus Sutra which he'd read for years, where vast numbers of *bodhisattvas* spring from the ground when Buddha is in need of help. That image had helped Sugiura grasp what a hellish situation Yoshida had been in. Seeing this on the Internet, Sugiura had been reminded how typical this was of Yoshida.

"It was just like Yoshida to think like that and to see his staff risking their lives to get the situation under control. That analogy to the *bodhisattvas* is a really good image. His staff came back to the plant, despite their exhaustion, to resume their efforts to contain the problem. When Buddha summoned them, it was to help spread his doctrine, but the image of countless *bodhisattvas* erupting from the ground must have corresponded with that of his staff, confronting the catastrophe with indomitable courage. *That was impressive*, I'd thought. That's how Yoshida would perceive his staff, and exactly how he'd express the situation. It makes you appreciate his consideration and compassion for his trusted employees."

Another of Yoshida's classmates from high school days visited FDI after the accident. This was Hajime Taniguchi, head of the Takenaka Research & Development Institute.

"From my point of view, in high school Yoshida was a tough young man, and gave a bit of a scary impression. He became an executive officer at TEPCO and I heard that at board meetings he could be really outspoken and blunt. In 2010 he came to tell me he was being sent to be superintendent at FDI, and I replied something about that being tough."

Of course Taniguchi had no idea what troubles awaited Yoshida there.

"Our corporation has a nuclear power section, so when Units 1, 3 and 4 exploded, we got the job of making covers for them. We were assigned the work on Unit 4, and by e-mail, Yoshida invited me to visit him just once, so I took my team with me. It was in November, eight months after the accident. We all dressed up in Tyveks and boot covers, the works. Yoshida was waiting to meet us at the QPB. I was impressed to see the uniform of the national women's soccer team, Nadeshiko Japan, displayed near the video-conference screen. It belonged to Aya Sameshima, who played in the team that won the World Cup. Yoshida gleefully explained that it was their lucky charm. The TEPCO Mareeze women's soccer team was based in Fukushima, and Yoshida was friendly with some of the players. During the Beijing Olympics, I had a meeting in Tokyo with Yoshida on the very day Nadeshiko had a match. I invited him to the party after the meeting, but he declined saying he was sorry but he'd go straight home; there was a match he just had to watch. He was a stalwart supporter of women's soccer. After the accident, when the Japanese women's team won the World Cup, it must have given him a real boost."

After graduating from high school, Yoshida went on to the Tokyo Institute of Technology, where he joined the rowing club. Keiji Nagano, now a researcher at Honda R&D, was one of his fellow rowers.

"Yoshida and I were always together in the rowing club. The largest boat, the eight, carries nine people including the cox, but all the rowers face the stern, so only the cox can see where you're going. Yoshida and I were in the center four seats, the engine, with me in the fourth seat from the bow, and him in the fifth, so I always rowed facing his back. Yoshida wasn't just the tallest in our year but had long legs with it, so we had trouble getting our timing right at first.You don't row these boats with your arms so much as with your legs, you know. When you wear trousers, the thighs are always close to bursting because your legs build up a lot muscle. We'd get up at four-thirty every morning. And lights-out was at eight-thirty, so we'd joke about when we were supposed to do our homework. The boathouse was at Toda in Saitama so we used to camp out there. We'd usually practice on the Toda Rowing Course and sometimes go out on the Arakawa River, come back to the boathouse, shower off together and then head for school. We'd be so sleepy that the lessons were pretty much a waste of time. Of course, Yoshida was a bit different from everybody else. He knew a lot about religious topics and once, when we had new eights built, he decided names for each of them. Being up on religion and Chinese stuff, he used the names of fictional creatures from Chinese mythology. I remember he named one of them *Taihō*, after a gigantic fish that changed into an equally enormous bird. This *Taihō* could cover ninety thousand leagues in a single flap of its wings. We used to wonder how on earth he knew things like that. He certainly had his own special kind of atmosphere. Later, he was even accepted for a position at METI, the Ministry of Economy, Trade and Industry, but turned it down to go to TEPCO."

Having spent his post-graduate years on theory and research into atomic nuclei, he chose a career not with the ministry that governed nuclear power but with a company that actually operated and maintained nuclear power stations.

Back to the ERC

Yoshida and his wife, Yōko, had met at college, and married in 1980, a year after he joined TEPCO.

"He'd been reading books on religion since he was young, so I've often felt he had an air of the temple about him. Whenever we go on trips and we visit a famous temple, he usually persuades the resident priest to show him around behind the scenes. He's a bit pushy that way. But seeing how he handled things like that made me see him as very mature. Ever since he was young he's been different from his contemporaries. I think he has always had a bit of a preoccupation with life and death. When I think of death myself, it's something fearful, but he has a more philosophical attitude, so I don't think he views death the same way. He has this unusual outlook on life and death, and seems to think that if you die it's not something to worry about, and hearing him talk about it has been a great relief to me at times. He takes things as they come. He doesn't believe in making a fuss about things. I suppose he has always had a fatalistic kind of attitude like that."

Eight months after the accident, Yoshida was suddenly diagnosed with esophageal cancer. Having battled on against enormous stress, his body was suddenly being eroded.

"He took the cancer announcement the same way. The examination he'd undergone at the TEPCO hospital had revealed a large shadow around his esophagus, and he was sent to Keio University Hospital for a detailed follow up. The results came back on November sixteenth. The doctor explained that it was a Stage III cancer of the esophagus, but both of us listened as dispassionately as if the patient were somebody else. I suppose we'd already detached ourselves, and the doctor's voice seemed to be coming from far, far away. It wasn't until much, much later that I began to feel more emotional and wonder why my husband was being treated so cruelly after he had tried so hard."

For someone who had so gallantly walked the line between life and death, it was a bitter fate. In order to undergo more detailed tests he needed to stay in hospital, so he handed over the reins of FDI to his successor, Takeshi Takahashi.

At the beginning of December he was able to return to FDI, and visited the scene of his long battle, the emergency response center in the quakeproof building, to greet his assembled former subordinates.

Hundreds of people, including many from the contractors, had squeezed into the ERC for another glimpse of Yoshida, who had disappeared from the plant so suddenly. He took the microphone and stood in front of the video-conference screen to address the assembly.

"Good to see you, everybody!" he began.

Since the plant was still contaminated, everyone wore Tyvek suits, even indoors. If you went one step outside the building, you needed to wear a full-face mask.

"I must apologize profoundly for handing over to Takahashi like this without even saying goodbye. As I'm sure you've already heard, the doctors have diagnosed my condition as Stage III cancer of the esophagus."

In the jam-packed ERC, the staff who had battled the reactors with him stifled their reactions in order not to miss a word.

"I'm scheduled to undergo chemotherapy and an operation. The doctors say that if they remove the affected part, I'll recover, so I'm going to leave matters in their hands. After working here with you all, I'm extremely sorry to leave you all in a situation like this. It's a real gut-wrencher," Yoshida announced to these people who'd worked under him, remembering the incredible hardships they'd faced together.

"I will never forget those days. The situation is still grim, but it's thanks to you that we were somehow able to get this far."

They listened to him and recalled their own trials, both Yoshida's own employees and contractor personnel alike. The atmosphere began to grow a little somber, so Yoshida produced one of his famous jokes. Mentioning the name of one of his balding senior staff, he gleefully announced, "I've had one round of chemical treatment, but my hair hasn't started falling out yet. Even after the treatment, look, I've still got more on top than *he* has!"

Immediately, with a roar of laughter, everyone's eyes flipped back and forth, comparing his hair with that of the chief of General Affairs standing at the edge of the crowd. Typical Yoshida.

"I want you all to carry on here. There are still difficulties to overcome but I know you'll do your best to handle them. The people of Fukushima, and the whole nation, have their hopes on you. Never forget that. I want to see you pull together under Takahashi's leadership. Thank you for everything. I'll be back one day."

The end of his emotion-filled farewell greeting was followed by thunderous applause that filled the ERC.

"Thank you very much!"
"Hang in there!"
"Get well and come back soon!"

As he left the room, the staff crowded close to call out their own last words. Some were weeping. It was the farewell of fellow soldiers who had fought a hard battle together.

Yoshida commented: "They all crowded around when I left, you know. Calling out to me. They were obviously concerned. Until then, they'd not been told much about my condition, and at first, nobody really wanted to talk about it, I hear. But when they got it from the horse's mouth, with a few jokes thrown in, they seemed to be relieved. I was embarrassed at abandoning them like that, but they were all excited. Since the accident, there were no women there, because they aren't allowed to work in a radioactive environment, but there were plenty of people who wanted to shake my hand."

After that Yoshida headed for the Fukushima Daini plant.

"I went to FDN and visited the QPB there to make my farewells. A number of my men were exposed to radiation up to the permissible limit while responding to the accident. I had sent them to the newly created Stabilization Center at FDN and told them to work on the support side, so now they were working there. So there were crowds of my own men who'd gathered to see me there. The room was packed with them, and when it was time to leave they gave me a very cheering send-off."

So it was that Yoshida bid farewell to his comrades in arms.

Chernobyl times ten

On February 7, 2012, Yoshida had been through an operation for his esophageal cancer, and though the subsequent chemotherapy caused him to suffer from vomiting and gagging, he was making a recovery. However, on February 26 he suffered a brain hemorrhage, requiring two open surgeries and a catheter operation. His convalescence was no holiday.

His wife Yōko explained: "The operation for his cancer was a big one, requiring the removal of a rib and taking nearly ten hours. He came out of hospital for a while but then collapsed with a brain hemorrhage. Seeing him in that state made me ask myself why he had to suffer like this. I seriously began to wonder if the gods hated him. And after Papa had worked so hard! But the fact that a man like him had been in Fukushima when he was needed was fate, I realized. I asked myself, *Out of all of Japan's one hundred and thirty million people, why did Papa have to be the one chosen?*, but then realized that ever since he was young he'd talked about accepting his fate, and I thought all this must have been destiny. He never complained about it in front of me, so I don't really know, but after the accident, when he had had to decide who would be sent home and who would stay, there were lots of women and young people in the QPB at the time. It must have been heartbreaking for him."

Site Superintendent Yoshida had kindly answered my questions during the short period in July 2012 between his cancer operation and when he collapsed with a brain hemorrhage. The thing that remained most vividly in my own mind from the long hours of the interview was his description of what he foresaw as the worst-case scenario. The one thing that he could never shake from his mind was the sheer scale of the problem that had landed on his shoulders.

"If the containment vessel ruptured, contamination would be spread far and wide, and the radiation levels would make it impossible to approach the plant. That would make it impossible to cool any of the reactors. Humans would no longer be able to do anything to the reactors. The plant at FDN, too, would become unapproachable, which – when you think about exactly how many reactor cores would be melting down (with FDI and FDN, that's a total of ten reactors destroyed) – so, as a rough estimate, that would make it ten times as big as Chernobyl. That was the thing that really weighed on my mind as I tried to handle the situation. That was what was so amazing about the personnel at the plant. To prevent that worst-case scenario, they repeatedly went into the reactor buildings, right up until the end. Then there were masses of other brave people I'd like to pay tribute to, starting with the Self Defense Forces, who came without regard for their own lives to help at the plant. Though the accident inflicted enormous damage on the people of Fukushima, I'm lost for words to express my gratitude to those who fought so bravely to prevent an even worse outcome."

Yoshida had told me that the worst-case scenario was ten times as big as Chernobyl. When I told Madaramé of the Nuclear Safety Commission what Yoshida had told me, this was his response:

"Yoshida went as far as that, did he? I really admire those people at the plant. The worst-case scenario that I envisaged could have been even worse than what Yoshida foresaw. There are more nuclear power plants nearby besides FDN. If FDI had gone completely out of control then, not only FDN but the Tokai No.2 Power Station in Ibaraki would have been knocked out too. If that had happened, the country might well have been divided into three: the uninhabitable contaminated area, the northern island of Hokkaido, and the rest of western Japan. Split into three pieces, it would have been the end for Japan."

The continued injection of water, even when it seemed as if the end had come, had finally ended the reactors' rampage. Though the people of Fukushima and the surrounding areas had suffered enormous damage, it is safe to say that the selfless efforts of those at the site had prevented even greater losses.

Masao Yoshida, who, with his team, had faced this unprecedented nuclear accident, had finally arrived at the conclusion of that major role and now faced a new battle, for his own health.

Epilogue

Saturday, November 26, 2011

Almost nine months had passed since the earthquake. With no end to the contamination in sight, life as an evacuee dragged on.

The nuclear refugees were occasionally allowed to visit their former homes inside the twenty-kilometer evacuation zone, but the dilapidated condition of the abandoned houses was a terrible shock to the owners. With no human interference, the weeds had invaded unrestrained, and the well-loved scenes they remembered had been transformed into a painfully pitiful imitation.

Every time Ikuo Izawa, the head of the control room for Units 1 and 2 at FDI, saw such scenes broadcast on TV, his heart ached.

As a refugee himself, his own circumstances were little different from those of the families appearing in the TV programs. Two weeks or so after Site Superintendent Yoshida had departed the FDI plant suffering from esophageal cancer, Izawa was at the Hotel Listel Inawashiro, which enjoys views over Lake Inawashiro and west towards Mt Bandai.

The forty or so residents of Izawa's neighborhood, who had been scattered far and wide, had assembled for the first time since the accident.

The organizers had invited everyone to the overnight get-together to see all the old faces and find out how everyone was getting along. The other topic was how they were going to face their uncertain future.

It wasn't even December, but it had already snowed in the area around Lake Inawashiro. On Friday, temperatures in the region had fallen to minus 0.1°C, and snow had started to flurry. Even the maximum temperature that day was only 1.5°C, and the snow that started to fall in the afternoon had turned the world into a frosted fairyland. Mt Bandai (1,816 meters) to the west from the hotel, was vaguely visible, but was clearly dressed in its winter robes, floating above the magical scene. Saturday, however, turned sunny and in the afternoon the temperature rose to a far-more-comfortable five degrees, making the previous day's snow seem like a dream.

Izawa had brought his eighty-six-year-old father with him in his car, all the way from Iwaki.

He had only decided to take part in the event after considerable debate.

His father, born in 1926, (the last year of the reign of the emperor Taishō), didn't have much time left. *If we skip this,* he thought, *Dad may never get to meet his old friends and neighbors again.* That was what persuaded him to bring his father to the gathering.

At the same time, it would be the first time since the disaster for Izawa to face the people among whom he had grown up, all of whom knew he was a TEPCO employee. He racked his brains thinking about how to address, how to even face these people who had been driven from their homes into the tribulations of refugeehood. How on earth could he apologize to them?

The problem obsessed him. He'd consider himself lucky if he got away with nothing more than a few rude shouts and jeers, he thought. He wanted to listen to their resentment and complaints with his own ears, and make a sincere apology. There were so many to whom since his childhood he had become indebted, and he had come intending to meet them face to face and open his heart to them.

"Hey, Ikuo-*chan*!"

As he entered the hotel lobby with his father, just by chance, someone noticed him and rushed to his side, addressing him with his given name and the term "*-chan*", used when addressing children, close friends and family.

"Ikuo-*chan*, are you all right? You must have had a hard time."

People came up to greet him, people who'd come all the way here from Aizu, Fukushima, Tokyo, even Chiba. And they addressed this man of over fifty as "Ikuo-*chan*"! These were people who knew him better than anyone, and had done so since he had enjoyed the fruits of the land and the sea in his boyhood days in Fukushima's Hamadōri.

Izawa was lost for words.

Deep in the back of his mind, scenes of the days spent as he and his men held out in the darkness of the control room began to replay. The colleagues who had gone on the endless visits to the turbine building and who had made the desperate incursions into the reactor building reappeared before him. They too were local men, all from Fukushima.

In the evening there was a dinner party in the hotel's banquet room. Though the room was grand, the members of the party all came from a community of only twenty households or so. There were barely forty participants. It was rather a large room for the number of people.

Izawa's father was led to the seats at the front reserved for the most senior members, while Izawa selected the most inconspicuous seat he could find at the back.

The master of ceremonies, over eighty years old himself, took the stage, microphone in hand.

His heartfelt opening speech rang through the room, commending them all for the way they had dealt with the hardships they had gone through since the disaster. Now they needed to continue to support each other, he told them. Then, as he approached the end of his address, the MC started to speak with the intonation peculiar to the local dialect.

"As some of you will already know, I am ever-so-glad to be able to tell you that today we have been joined by none other than our very own Ikuo-*chan*!"

Izawa gulped. He'd intended to stay out of sight, but now the MC was referring to him from the stage.

"I know things haven't worked out very well," he noted preliminarily, with respect to their mutual situation. "But, Ikuo-*chan* has been doing his best. Right to the end . . .

"To protect our community, he remained at his post, right to the end. And our dear Ikuo-*chan* has come here today especially to see all of us!"

As he spoke his eyes shifted to Izawa, right at the back. Of course, the eyes of the whole party followed.

Izawa froze. He was unable to move. The MC took a breath and continued.

"For Ikuo-*chan*, who stuck to his post right to the very end, may I call for a round of applause?"

Izawa was dumbstruck.

The next moment a wave of applause swept the room. It was enormous.

Everyone had turned to face him and was clapping.

"Thank you, Ikuo-*chan*!" they called. These people, who had been banished from their ancestral homes and thrown into the deprived life of refugees, who had suffered so much already, continued to applaud and thank him.

These people who had known Ikuo-*chan* since he was a child could imagine full well how hard he had tried to protect their community. This applause came from people who knew him well enough to understand, without being told, that Ikuo-*chan* would undoubtedly have done his absolute best.

In spite of himself, Izawa's eyes filled with tears.

He stood.

He had to make some kind of apology, even if it was only a few words. And then he must thank them for such a warm welcome despite the circumstances.

But Izawa was no longer able to speak. Tears streamed down his cheeks and splashed on the floor.

All he could do was stand and hang his head. Thoughts of his home-town and his gratitude to the people who had shared it with him filled him, and robbed him of the power of speech.

Thank you, thank you. . . .

Though in his heart the words were repeated over and over, they never reached his mouth. The applause rang on and on as his eighty-six-year-old father, born in another era, looked on in silence.

Conclusion

When I called on Shūrō Shiga, the former mayor of Ōkuma and a living witness to the history of FDI from its birth until the catastrophe, it was the beginning of August 2012, seventeen months after the earthquake.

The eighty-year-old was living as a refugee in an apartment in southern Fukushima. Having lost most of his sight in a failed operation several years previously, the only visual images he retained were lively ones of the days when it was his home.

Shūrō's father, Hidemasa, had become mayor of Ōkuma in 1962 and had devoted his energies to wooing the power plant to the area. Shiga the younger had himself been mayor from September 1987 to September 2007 and had worked to revitalize the area.

The two of them had, in effect, brought nuclear power to Ōkuma and maintained the balance that enabled the town to coexist with the plant, such that their whole lives were spent connected to the nuclear industry. At the same time, Shiga the younger, who could remember all the ups and downs since the pre-war years, was a living witness.

"When that area became the Iwaki Army Airbase, I was in elementary school. We were the nearest house to the airfield, so when it went into operation, one of the flying instructors used to have his 'digs' at our place. Bed and board, it was. Sometimes the instructor would bring candy or chewing gum, and I often got some for myself. He said he wanted to ride a horse, so I took our farmhorse to the airfield. The airstrip was all turf, and enormous. Five or six soldiers gathered around and had fun horse-riding. Well, it was wartime and there wasn't much else in the way of fun to be had. I remember we often used to see the *Red Dragonfly* trainer biplanes there on our way home from school."

When the war ended, Shiga was in his second year at Futaba junior high.

"After the war, that place was used as saltpans. In those days, the only place in Japan where they made salt was down south near the Seto Inland Sea. There was a salt shortage, so Kokudo Keikaku got in there and built their Iwaki Salt Works."

Kokudo was under the wing of Yasujirō Tsutsumi (a notorious politician, convicted, along with about one hundred and fifty others, of election offences after his twelfth re-election in 1963.) As a politician, he had all right the connections in government for branching out into a new business, because until 2002, salt was a controlled substance, regulated by the Ministry of Finance. He built pools up there on the hill. Then they built frames covered in bamboo branches and splashed seawater over them, letting evaporation produce the salt. After a few years of that, the chemical industry developed easier ways to make salt and the saltpan industry was abandoned."

Later the state-owned land was distributed to private owners.

"Everyone planted pine trees on their properties. When the trees were five or six meters tall, *amitake,* a popular kind of edible mushroom, known in English as the Jersey cow mushroom, would appear around the bottom of the trunks. You could just wander around and collect whole basketfuls of the stuff, so everyone would be out there. Talk of building the power station there didn't come until much later."

The first step was taken in the late 1950s, when a survey was carried out to assess the water quality.

"When the army airfield was there, we had enough that we used to pump water and pipe it out there to them for their drinking water. So in the late fifties, when they started planning the reactors, they came to our place to sample the water. My father became mayor in November of '62, and he thought if they could get the plant built there, the local people would no longer have to traipse around the country looking for seasonal work every winter, which would bring prosperity to the community and the whole area. Bringing prosperity to the area was the goal in his mind. But it was still only seventeen years since the nuclear bombs of Hiroshima and Nagasaki, and that memory was still fresh. But we in the community didn't know anything about how nuclear power really worked. If the national and prefectural government said it was safe, we'd believe them. That's why there was no organized opposition to the project."

Shiga's wife, Tsuneko, recalls how, once construction began, a girl from the GE village often came to their house to play.

"Our second girl became friends with her. The house wasn't far off, so she'd often come over to play. We had this big Japanese doll, which we gave to her. Then, every time she came to play, she happily brought that doll with her. The doll was one of those dress-up kinds where you can change the kimonos. The girl hadn't started school, but she took great care of it. She'd bring us big bars of chocolate too, and before they went back to the States, she somehow managed to tell my daughter she was going home."

In 1987, Shiga the younger was elected mayor of Ōkuma, and as demand for electric power rose, so did the status of nuclear plants.

"As you'd expect, with the construction of the plant, the area began to change. The winding lanes were turned into straight, asphalted roads, the contour-running rice paddies re-organized into efficient rectangles. Under the *Dengen Sampō*, three new laws for power source development, there was new funding available. All kinds of things were improved. What with property taxes on the nuclear-related facilities and the like, the town was much better off. When my father worked in the finance department around 1950, the town coffers were empty, and I was repeatedly sent to borrow money from the wealthier local families. That's how poor Ōkuma was in those days. But with the coming of the nuclear plant, things really improved. While I was mayor, we made health care completely free up to junior high school age and our sanitation rates were the cheapest in the country. We did all kinds of things to bring prosperity to the community. But in the end, it all turned out like this."

This was how the eighty-year old, living far from his hometown as a refugee in an apartment, retraced the history of FDI. In the end, they had not only lost their homes in Ōkuma, but were completely banished from the area.

Having devoted his whole career to improving the area, Shiga must have felt that his whole life's work had been wasted. During our interviews he often sighed deeply. Though he wasn't so uncouth as to put it into words himself, the sighs, along with the deep lines in his face, made it clear that the accident at TEPCO, the company that had so completely won their trust, was an unbearable burden to him.

Makoto Kamino, former head of the Tomioka branch of the regional newspaper *Fukushima Minpō*, who had driven from Tomioka to Kawauchi village to continue reporting after the evacuation area was enlarged the day after the accident, is one who knows full well the local people's dismay with TEPCO. He feels that the depth of their former trust in TEPCO has only amplified the present anger and despair in the local community.

"It was on March twenty-third that the vice president of TEPCO visited the multipurpose convention facilities in Kōriyama city known as Big Palette Fukushima, where the evacuees from Tomioka and Kawauchi were being sheltered, and went around apologizing to each of them. While he was there, someone spoke up and said, 'Everyone else is being polite and not mentioning it, but since it's nothing to do with me, I can tell you what these people *really* think. What the hell are you doing here NOW? You're too damn late!' To be frank, I think he summed up the anger of the betrayed community precisely. TEPCO had truly blended into the community. There were some married employees who had been posted to Tomioka unaccompanied, but many had brought their families. They weren't there just on company orders; they really had settled down there and won the trust of the local people. I grew up in Fukushima city myself, so I only discovered how strong this feeling was when I came to work at the Tomioka office. This made all the more reason for these people whose town had been made uninhabitable, to feel betrayed by TEPCO."

The unforeseen nuclear disaster brought on by the tsunami has left deep scars in other places too.

As I continued my research for this book, I was made painfully aware of the numerous lessons in a variety of subjects that this nuclear accident has left for future generations. These lessons are relevant not only to the world of nuclear power, but are aphorisms that I think are applicable to several fields.

Also, while paying homage to those who labored within the

plant, it is difficult to avoid reaching the conclusion that the politicians, the administration, TEPCO – those responsible for the management and promotion of nuclear power, but who nevertheless failed to prevent the accident – were guilty of conceit.

There were two opportunities when the disaster could have been forestalled. The more significant of them was September 11, 2001.

It should hardly need repeating that the two major 'enemies' of nuclear power, – against which in the interest of safety, double and triple defenses are installed – are natural disasters and terrorism.

The largest factor in the disaster at FDI, the overreliance placed on the ten-meter height difference between the plant and sea-level, falls under the category of natural disasters.

"No tsunami would reach ten meters above sea level."

This preconception was an underestimate, a naïve trust in the forces of nature, instilled by a thousand years without a large tsunami in Hamadōri.

But there is no guarantee that future natural disasters will fall within the range of past ones. Such a belief is mere wishful thinking.

It is also a measure of man's arrogance toward the forces of nature. The event that should have warned against such arrogance was the 9-11 terrorist attack by followers of Osama bin Laden.

Bin Laden's attack was not a natural disaster. His attack was without question an act of terror. But this catastrophe, with its almost three thousand deaths, was also a clear warning to nuclear power. It warned us that terrorist attacks of unprecedented scale were the greatest threat to the nuclear industry. The US nuclear industry responded quickly.

Measures against terrorism were immediately strengthened, and the question of how to control a reactor if there were a complete station blackout was debated with renewed vigor.

Five years later, in 2006, the United States Nuclear Regulatory Commission produced a series of enhancements to the existing emergency preparedness regulations and guidance, which were forwarded to Japan.

The documents included precise details of procedures for the manual operation of a station under complete blackout, including the provision and location of portable compressors and batteries.

The nuclear power station's Achilles' heel with regard to both terrorist attacks and natural disasters is that of loss of power, in that it means the loss of ability to cool the reactors.

Nevertheless, for the nuclear power plants of Japan, the foreseeable consequences of a total loss of power and subsequent inability to cool the reactors were not even among the hypothetical emergency conditions examined.

That kind of terrorism couldn't happen in Japan! people thought.

Despite the fact that certain neighboring countries have missiles aimed at Japan, this baseless presumption seemed like an infection that had spread even among the leaders who control and promote nuclear energy. But the natural disaster that *did* strike was at least as bad, if not worse than what any terrorist might have done. It may be a harsh and even vulgar term, but I think the often-heard phrase 'drunk with peace' is appropriate here.

In my own opinion, the immature and optimistic assumption by the leaders of the government bodies responsible for nuclear power, and even the heads of the nuclear industry, that Japan alone among the nations of the world is a target neither for terrorism, nor for missile attack, is proof that they are incompetent. I am dismayed that scenarios of terrorism or military conflict leading to complete loss of power, or of the ability to cool the reactors, are not even considered. If, like the US, they had taken even a few measures, the procedures for avoiding complete loss of power or cooling capacity would at least have been considered, avoiding much of the damage brought about by this natural disaster. But that opportunity was lost.

The other opportunity came three years and three months after 9-11 with the Sumatra Earthquake of December 26, 2004. The M9.3 quake and the huge tsunami it roused took two hundred and twenty thousand lives and literally shook the whole world. Together, they showed that nature could exceed human imagination.

Needless to say, precautions against such eventualities as complete loss of power or cooling capacity have a price. Nuclear power operators exist to make a profit, so difficult decisions need to be made.

In effect, both the government and the industry chose profit over safety. This attitude shows a lack of due respect for the incredible forces unleashed by this human invention, nuclear power. Here, in the only country ever to have suffered a nuclear attack, I cannot find words to describe its leaders' alarming apathy.

It didn't become general knowledge until twenty years later, in 2012, that in 1992 the Nuclear Safety Commission had declared that it was not necessary to evaluate the scenario of a complete power loss of more than thirty minutes, and had deferred the revision of its safety principles. As Haruki Madaramé, head of the Nuclear Safety Commission, observed regretfully at the press conference to mark the replacement of the commission by a new Nuclear Regulation Authority, "Effectively, the problem of whether or not nuclear safety can be maintained depends on human beings."

Surely this is the essence of the matter.

Thanks to the last-ditch efforts of the people inside the plant, Yoshida's worst case of 'Chernobyl times ten' was avoided by a hair's breadth. However, as is now common knowledge, it will be a very long time indeed before Fukushima and its surroundings can be restored, and meanwhile the refugees are still suffering.

While the tremendous energy of the anti-nuclear movement that arose after the accident is only to be expected, I am deeply apprehensive at the sudden disappearance of voices condemning the thermal power stations that contribute significantly to global warming and other forms of environmental damage. Instead of being swept away in this flood of extremism, Japan, a land of limited natural resources, needs its people to sit down calmly and apply every bit of its intellectual resources to finding a way to make ends meet until the country can be sustained by renewable energy.

Chronology

Year	Date	Event
1939	June	3,000 hectares on the coastal hills of Ottozawa in the village of Kuma-machi bought by compulsory purchase order for the construction of an army airbase.
1941	April	Iwaki branch of the army's Utsunomiya Flying School opened. Equipped with Type 95 "Red Dragonfly" intermediate training aircraft (US designation Tachikawa Ki-9 "Spruce").
1945	Feb	Training carried out for "special attack" pilots. Many young men left here destined to become kamikaze pilots.
	Aug 9~10	Airfield destroyed by two days of concentrated US Navy bombardment.
	Aug 15	Military control ceases with the armistice.
1948		Kokudo develops the area as saltpans.
1956	Jan 1	*Dengen Sampō,* three Acts concerning nuclear power, come into effect.
1957	Feb 22	The nine electric power companies settle their plan for nuclear power.
1960	May 10	Fukushima prefecture joins the Japan Atomic Industrial Forum.
	Nov 29	Fukushima prefecture offers TEPCO a site in Futaba for development of a nuclear power station.

1961	Sept	With the assent of the town councils of Ōkuma and Futaba, the respective mayors confirm their invitation to TEPCO to build a nuclear power station.
1964	Dec 1	TEPCO sets up a survey station in Ōkuma.
1966	April 4	A Boiling Water Reactor from GE is chosen as the first unit at FDI.
	Dec 2	Construction starts on Unit 1.
1969	April 4	Fukushima prefecture and TEPCO sign an agreement on ensuring safety at the nuclear power plant.
	May 27	Construction starts on Unit 2.
1970	July 4	First insertion of fuel assemblies into Unit 1.
	Oct 17	Construction starts on Unit 3.
	Nov 17	First test run of Unit 1 starts.
1971	March 26	Unit 1 commences business operation.
	Dec 22	Construction starts on Unit 5.
1972	Sept 12	Construction starts on Unit 4.
1973	May 18	Construction starts on Unit 6.
	June 25	Waste liquid leaks from a radioactive liquid waste storage tank. A 22-hour delay in informing Ōkuma town council causes a crisis.
1974	July 18	Unit 2 commences business operation.
1976	March 27	Unit 3 commences business operation.
1978	April 18	Unit 5 commences business operation.
	Oct 12	Unit 4 commences business operation.
1979	March 28	Nuclear accident at Three Mile Island.
	Oct 24	Unit 6 commences business operation.
1986	April 26	Nuclear accident at Chernobyl.

Year	Date	Event
2007	July 16	Earthquake occurs off Niigata coast at 10:13. (Niigataken Chūetsu-oki Earthquake) Intensity level 6+ observed at Kashiwazaki city. Active reactor units 2, 3, 4, and 7 at the TEPCO Kashiwazaki-Kariya nuclear plant automatically shutdown safely. Electrical fire occurs in the Unit 3 reactor building but is extinguished by the local fire brigade at 12:10.
2010	July 20	Quakeproof emergency response building opened at Fukushima Daiichi.
2011	March 11	Great East Japan Earthquake (M9) occurs off Fukushima coast at 14:46. At 15:41, tsunami causes station blackout.
	March 12	Hydrogen explosion at Unit 1. Seawater injected into Unit 1 reactor. 20 km compulsory evacuation zone declared.
	March 13	Unit 3 loses cooling functions. Fire engines inject seawater.
	March 14	Hydrogen explosion at Unit 3. Containment vessel at Unit 2 exceeds maximum operating pressure.
	March 15	Explosion heard at Unit 2. Suppression chamber loses all pressure. Explosion and fire at Unit 4 reactor building. Inhabitants in the 20 to 30 km zone are told to stay indoors.
	March 16	Fire at Unit 4. White smoke seen coming from Unit 3.
	March 17	JGSDF helicopters drop water into spent fuel pools at Unit 3. Simultaneously, JGSDF and JASDF fire engines conduct hosing operations from the ground.
	March 18	Installation of power lines commences. Units 1, 2 and 3 events upgraded to INES level 5. (Unit 4: level 4)
	March 19	Tokyo fire brigade hoses spent fuel pool at Unit 3.
	March 22	External power sources restored at all six reactors.
	March 26	1,000 mSv/h detected at Unit 2 turbine building.
	April 2	Highly contaminated water detected leaking into the sea near the Unit 2 seawater inlet.
	April 4	10,000 tons of low-level contaminated water released into the sea from the radioactive waste disposal facility.

2011	April 6	Coagulant polymer injected into the ground successfully stops high-level waste water leak.
	April 7	Nitrogen injected into Unit 1 containment vessel.
	April 11	External power source cut off by further tremors. Water injection for Units 1, 2 and 3 temporarily halted.
	April 12	INES Level raised to 7, the same as Chernobyl.
	April 17	TEPCO announces first schedule for recovery.
	April 22	The 20 km zone is declared a restricted area. Surrounding area warned to be ready to evacuate. Entry restrictions applied.
	May 11	Highly contaminated water leaks into the sea from Unit 3.
	May 15	TEPCO confirms a meltdown at Unit 1.
	May 24	IAEA inspects FDI. TEPCO confirms meltdowns at Units 2 and 3.
	June 27	A cooling system recycling processed water into the reactor core goes into operation at Unit 3
	June 30	Cooling system started in the Unit 3 spent fuel pool.
	July 6	Government announces stress test for all reactors.
	Aug 10	Recycling cooling system in operation for all spent fuel pools at Units 1 to 4.
	Aug 31	TEPCO announces decommissioning schedule. Proposal to flood containment vessel with water while fuel rods are removed.
	Sept 19	At the IAEA general meeting, Gōshi Hosono, minister in charge of the accident, vows to achieve cold shutdown by the end of the year.
	Sept 20	Groundwater, up to 500 tons per day, found to be flowing into the basement of the reactor buildings.
	Sept 21	Water leaks from Unit 6 turbine building.
	Sept 28	Water in the base of the Unit 1, 2, and 3 pressure vessels brought below 100°C.
	Sept 30	Restrictions on the 20 to 30 km evacuation zone are lifted.
	Oct 3	Government estimates cost of decommissioning at 1.15 trillion yen (about 15 billion USD).
	Oct 28	NSC announces decommissioning will take at least 30 years

2011	Nov 12	TEPCO opens site for inspection for the first time since the accident. Site Superintendent Masao Yoshida gives press conference.
	Nov 14	1300 mSv/h recorded at first floor of Unit 3.
	Dec 1	Site Superintendent Yoshida takes medical leave for esophageal cancer. Nitrogen injection into reactor vessels of Units 1 to 3 commences.
	Dec 2	TEPCO's investigation committee makes interim report.
	Dec 16	PM Noda announces that cold shutdown has been achieved, and the accident brought under control on schedule.
	Dec 18	Yūhei Satō, Governor of Fukushima prefecture, expresses displeasure at the PM's use of "brought under control." Environment Minister Hosono apologizes.
	Dec 21	TEPCO and the government announce it will be 10 years before they can start to remove the damaged fuel rods, and reveal a decommissioning schedule of up to 40 years.
	Dec 26	Government interim report stresses human failures and denies damage directly due to the earthquake.
2012	Jan 6	Government limits operational lifetime of all Japan's reactors to 40 years. It also reveals its "worst case scenario" as requiring evacuation of a 250 km zone including the Tokyo metropolis.
	Jan 28	Leaks detected from water decontamination facilities and injection pumps due to damage from freezing.
	Jan 31	The village of Kawauchi decides to return home, first among the surrounding municipalities. IAEA declares conditions safe, and the Diet passes the necessary legislation.
	Feb 10	Government establishes a Reconstruction Agency.
	Feb 13	Thermometer shows temperature rise in Unit 2 pressure vessel. TEPCO calls it a meter malfunction.
	Feb 28	RJIF (Rebuild Japan Initiative Foundation) publishes its independent report on the accident.
	March 11	Water leaks discovered in Unit 1 turbine building.

2012	March 26	Water level in Unit 2 containment vessel discovered to be only 60 cm.
	March 27	Intense radiation (72.9 Sv/h) observed at Unit 2.
	April 6	Ministry of Health, Labor and Welfare announced maximum exposure limits for workers in contaminated areas: 50 mSv/year and 100 mSv in 5 years.
	April 16	Compulsory and precautionary evacuation zones in Minami Sōma city deactivated.
	April 19	Units 1 to 4 officially scrapped under the Electricity Business Act.
	May 24	TEPCO estimates that the total release of radioactive material between March 12 and 31, 2011, amounted to 900,000 terabecquerels (TBq).
	June 20	TEPCO releases its final report on the accident.
	July 5	The Diet releases its independent report on the accident.
	July 23	The government committee on the accident hands in its final report.
	Aug 10	Almost the whole of the town of Naraha is removed from the restricted zone.
2013	July 9	Masao Yoshida dies.

Abbreviations and Terms

APD	Alarm Personal Dosimeters (APD)
AC	alternating current (like commercial grid power)
AM	Accident Management system
AO	Air Operated (valve)
BWR	Boiling Water Reactor
CBRN	Chemical, Biological, Radiological, and Nuclear
CR	control rods
DC	direct current (as from batteries)
DG	diesel generators
ECCS	Emergency Core Cooling System
ERC	emergency response center
FDI	Fukushima Daiichi
FDN	Fukushima Daiini
GE	General Electric Co.
GWe	gigawatts electrical
IAEA	International Atomic Energy Agency
INES	The International Nuclear and Radiological Event Scale
JASDF	Japanese Air Self-Defense Force
JCO	Japan Nuclear Fuel Conversion Office
JGSDF	Japanese Ground Self-Defense Force
JSDF	Japanese Self-Defense Force
kPa	kiloPascal, unit of pressure, 100 kPa≈1 atmosphere
Local HQ	Local Nuclear Emergency Response Headquarters
local intensity	Japanese "Shindo" scale of [earthquake intensity, i.e.] perceived local vibration. (Equivalent to the US Mercalli scale.)
LPCI	Low Pressure Coolant Injection
M9.0	magnitude 9.0, a measure of the energy released by the quake
METI	Ministry of Economy, Trade and Industry
MO	Motor Operated (valve)

MSIV	Main Steam Isolation Valve
mSv	milliSievert: measure of accumulated radiation
μSv	microSievert: measure of accumulated radiation
NERH	Nuclear Emergency Response Headquarters
NHK	Japan's national broadcasting corporation
NISA	Nuclear and Industrial Safety Agency
NRA	Nuclear Regulation Authority (formerly NSC)
NSC	Nuclear Safety Commission (now the Nuclear Regulation Authority)
OB	alumnus (old boy), also used to refer to people who have already retired from the company
Offsite Center	location of Local HQ, in Ōkuma
PA system	public address system
PCV	primary containment vessel
PMO	Prime Minister's Office
QPB	quakeproof building
RCIC	Reactor Core Isolation Cooling system
RHR	Residual Heat Removal
SBO	station black out
SCBA	self-contained breathing apparatus
Scram	emergency shutdown of the reactor
SRV	Safety Relief Valves
TEPCO	Tokyo Electric Power Company, Inc.
TEPCO HQ	TEPCO head office in Tokyo, Uchisawai-cho
Titech	Tokyo Institute of Technology
DRHQ	Tomioka's Disaster Response Headquarters
Tyvek®	anti-contamination suit
Unit 1	reactor #1 at FDI
μSv/h	microSieverts per hour: measure of radiation

Bibliography

Written in English, or official English translations:

ANS President's Special Committee on the Fukushima Accident – Report Summary. La Grange Park, IL, USA: American Nuclear Society, 2012.
http://www.fukushima.ans.org

Braun, Matthias. *The Fukushima Daiichi Incident*. Erlangen, Germany: AREVA–NP GmbH, 2011.
http://www.iaea.org/NuclearPower/Downloadable/Meetings/2011/2011-03-28-04-01-TWG-NPTD/Day3/FukushimaDaiichi-Braun-20110330.pdf

Executive summary report of the National Diet of Japan Fukushima Nuclear Accident Independent Investigation Commission, 2012. Tokyo: Fukushima Nuclear Accident Independent Investigation Commission, 2012.
http://www.nirs.org/fukushima/naiic_report.pdf
Source:『国会事故調報告書』（東京電力福島原子力発電所事故調査委員会）

Final Investigation Report of the Investigation Committee on the Accident at the Fukushima Nuclear Power Stations of Tokyo Electric Power Company, 2012. Tokyo: Investigation Committee on the Accident at the Fukushima Nuclear Power Stations, 2012.
http://www.cas.go.jp/jp/seisaku/icanps/eng/final-report.html
Source:『最終報告』（東京電力福島原子力発電所における事故調査・検証委員会）

Fukushima Daiichi Unit 1 Accident Timeline. La Grange Park, IL, USA: American Nuclear Society, 2012.
http://fukushima.ans.org/inc/Fukushima_Appendix_H.pdf

IAEA International Fact-Finding Expert Mission of the Fukushima Dai-ichi NPP Accident Following the Great East Japan Earthquake and Tsunami. Vienna, Austria: International Atomic Energy Agency, 2011.
http://www-pub.iaea.org/MTCD/meetings/PDFplus/2011/cn200/documentation/cn200_Final-Fukushima-Mission_Report.pdf

Interim Investigation Report of the Investigation Committee on the Accident at the Fukushima Nuclear Power Stations of Tokyo Electric Power Company, 2011. Tokyo: Investigation Committee on the Accident at the Fukushima Nuclear Power Stations, 2011.
http://www.cas.go.jp/jp/seisaku/icanps/eng/interim-report.html
Source:『中間報告』（東京電力福島原子力発電所における事故調査・検証委員会）

Japanese Earthquake and Tsunami: Implications for the UK Nuclear Industry, Final Report. London: HSE Office for Nuclear Regulation, 2011.
http://www.oecd-nea.org/nsd/fukushima/documents/UK_2011_10_final-ChiefInspectorreport.pdf

Linemann, Thomas & Mohrbach, Ludger. *The Accident at Fukushima.* Essen, Germany: VGB PowerTech Service GmbH, 2012.
http://www.elforsk.se/Global/Kärnkraft/filer/Dokumentation%202012/Linnemann_VGB.pdf

Report of the Fukushima Nuclear Accidents Investigation Committee, and attached materials. Tokyo: Tokyo Electric Power Co., Inc., 2011.
http://www.tepco.co.jp/en/press/corp-com/release/2012/1205638_1870.html
Source:『福島原子力事故調査報告書』及び『添付資料』（東京電力株式会社）

Report of the Independent Investigation Commission on the Fukushima Daiichi Nuclear Accident, and Rebuild Japan Initiative Foundation, 2012. Tokyo: Fukushima Daiichi Nuclear Accident Independent Investigation Commission, 2012.
http://warp.da.ndl.go.jp/info:ndljp/pid/3856371/naiic.go.jp/en/report/
Source:『福島原発事故独立検証委員会調査・検証報告書』（福島原発事故独立検証委員会・一般財団法人日本再建イニシアティブ）

Drawings and blueprints of special interest:

Attachment II-1, Overview of reactor facilities at the Fukushima Dai-ichi NPS
http://www.cas.go.jp/jp/seisaku/icanps/eng/120224Siryo02-1Eng.pdf
http://www.cas.go.jp/jp/seisaku/icanps/eng/120224Siryo02-2Eng.pdf

Written in Japanese:

大熊町史編纂委員会。『大熊町史第一巻〈通史〉』。大熊町、1985。(Ōkuma chōshi daiikkann (tsūshi); History of Ōkuma Town, Vol. 1). Ōkuma chōshi hensan iinkai, Ōkuma Town, 1985.

福山哲郎。『原発危機官邸からの証言』。東京：筑摩書房、2012。Fukuyama Tetsurō. (*Genpatsu kiki kantei kara no shōgen*; Testimony of the Prime Minister's Crisis Management Center). Tokyo: Chikuma Shobō, 2012.

細野豪志&鳥越俊太郎。『証言細野豪志』。講談社、2012。Hosono Gōshi and Torigoe Shuntarō, (*Shōgen hosono gōshi*; Testimony of Gōshi Hosono). Tokyo: Kōdansha, 2012.

日本戦没学生記念会。『きけわだつみのこえ』。日本戦没学生記念会、1995。(*Kiki wadatsumi no koe.* Nihon Senbotsu Gakusei Kinenkai, 1995). Portions translated in Moore, Aaron. *Writing War: Soldiers Record the Japanese Empire,* Harvard University Press, 2013.

All online documents were last accessed August 16, 2014.

A PDF of this bibliography with clickable URL links can be downloaded from:

https://www.kurodahan.com/wp/e/fukushima/

Contributors

Ryūshō Kadota (門田 隆将)

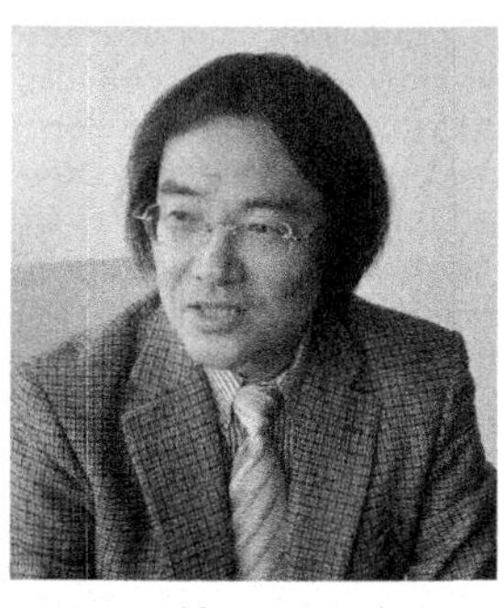

Born in Aki, Kochi Prefecture in 1958. After graduating Faculty of Law at Chūō University, entered Shinchōsha as a reporter at the Shūkan Shinchō weekly magazine, rising to assistant editor. After 7 years as a roving reporter, he wrote almost 800 articles during the 18 years he spent in the magazine's offices. He went independent in April 2008.

As a non-fiction author he is active in a wide range of genres including politics, law, crime, history, and sports, and has penned numerous books. *The Man Who Saved Taiwan: The Miracle of Lieutenant General Hiroshi Nemoto of the Imperial Japanese Army* (Kadokawa) was awarded the 19th Yamamoto Shichihei Prize. Other major books include *Kōshien Legacy: the Life of Legendary Batting Coach Michihiro Takabatake* (Kōdansha), *Battle Against Despair: The 3300 Days of Hiroshi Motomura* (Shinchōsha), *Last Testament of the Pacific War* (3 vols., Shōgakukan), and *Defanging the Wolf: The Tokyo Metropolitan Police Public Security Bureau and the Most Dangerous Bomber in Japan* (Shōgakukan).

Kōshien Legacy was dramatized by NHK as "Full Swing," starring Katsumi Takahashi, and *Battle Against Despair* was dramatized by WOWOW, starring Yōsuke Eguchi, winning the Grand Prize in the drama category at the National Arts Festival hosted by the Agency for Cultural Affairs.

His most recent work is *The Reporter Headed toward the Sea: The Tsunami, Radiation, and the Fukushima Minyū Shimbun* (Kadokawa). Kadota is continuing his dynamic writing in a wide range of fields.

http://www.kadotaryusho.com/

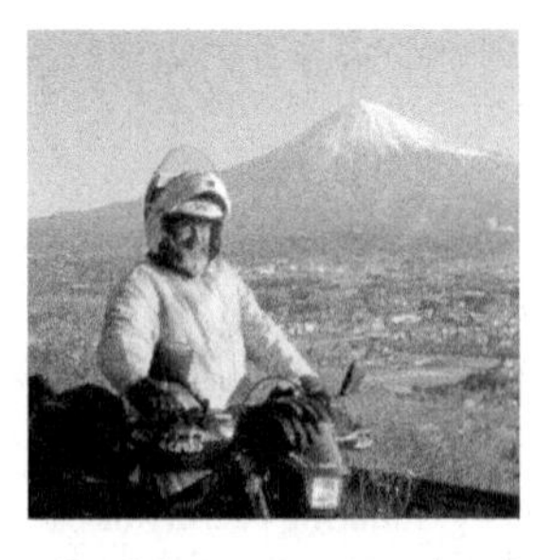

Simon Varnam was raised in a large family in the south of England on a diet of music, science fiction and walks in the country. He moved to Japan shortly after he finished college at Bangor, North Wales, where besides reading Physical Oceanography and Math he spent much effort on mountaineering and horn-playing. Having failed to become competent in French despite five years of study at secondary school, he was surprised to find that, thanks to complete immersion in the far north of the Tōhoku region, he picked up Japanese with relatively little effort. Twenty years later, he passed JLPT level 1 at first try and discovered the internet which led him to Japanese conservation organizations who needed English versions of their documents.

Since then he has translated (presentations, documents, articles, video subtitles and website pages) in a variety of fields; biodiversity and conservation, nuclear engineering, Japanese culture and an old love, science fiction. Simon now lives in the countryside at the foot of Mt Fuji with a Japanese wife, daughter and cat, and a garden full of wildlife.

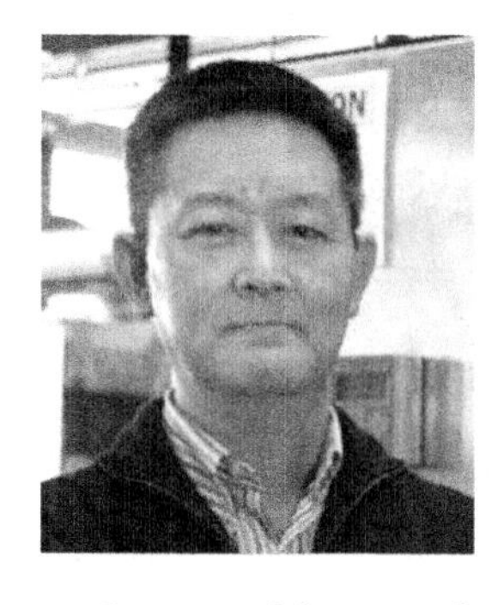

Akira Tokuhiro is Dean and Professor, Faculty of Energy Systems and Nuclear Science at University of Ontario Institute of Technology (Canada), known in short as "Ontario Tech". He was previously senior principle at NuScale Power, the small modular reactor startup that completed its design currently under review by the USNRC. He has been professor at University of Idaho, Kansas State University, University of Missouri – Rolla (UMR). At UMR, he was Director and licensed Senior Reactor Operator of the research reactor. He has diverse research interests centered around reactor engineering, next generation reactor concepts, safety, thermal hydraulics, experiments, modeling and simulation and complex phenomena. He served on the American Nuclear Society's President's Committee on the Fukushima Daiichi accident for 2011-2013. He also served on the Ontario Provincial Nuclear Emergency Response Plan review committee in 2017–2018.

Dr. Tokuhiro has 15+ years of international nuclear energy R&D and technology development experience in Canada, Switzerland and Japan. To date he has published 60+ papers, nearly 100 conference papers and worked with some 40 MS and PhD students. Although born in Tokyo, he was educated in the U.S. He holds a BSE, 1981, Engineering Physics, and PhD, 1991, Nuclear Engineering, both from Purdue University. He holds a MS, 1984, Mechanical Engineering, University of Rochester. He can be found on social media.

Printed in Great Britain
by Amazon